MW01253359

GUELPH HUMBER
205 Humber College Blvd
Toronto, ON   M9W 5L7

EMPATHY AND FAIRNESS

The Novartis Foundation is an international scientific and educational charity (UK Registered Charity No. 313574). Known until September 1997 as the Ciba Foundation, it was established in 1947 by the CIBA company of Basle, which merged with Sandoz in 1996, to form Novartis. The Foundation operates independently in London under English trust law. It was formally opened on 22 June 1949.

The Foundation promotes the study and general knowledge of science and in particular encourages international co-operation in scientific research. To this end, it organizes internationally acclaimed meetings (typically eight symposia and allied open meetings and 15–20 discussion meetings each year) and publishes eight books per year featuring the presented papers and discussions from the symposia. Although primarily an operational rather than a grant-making foundation, it awards bursaries to young scientists to attend the symposia and afterwards work with one of the other participants.

The Foundation's headquarters at 41 Portland Place, London W1B 1BN, provide library facilities, open to graduates in science and allied disciplines. Media relations are fostered by regular press conferences and by articles prepared by the Foundation's Science Writer in Residence. The Foundation offers accommodation and meeting facilities to visiting scientists and their societies.

Information on all Foundation activities can be found at http://www.novartisfound.org.uk

Novartis Foundation Symposium 278

16/10/

EMPATHY AND FAIRNESS

John Wiley & Sons, Ltd

Copyright © Novartis Foundation 2006
Published in 2007 by John Wiley & Sons Ltd,
      The Atrium, Southern Gate,
      Chichester PO19 8SQ, UK

      National   01243 779777
      International (+44) 1243 779777
      e-mail (for orders and customer service enquiries): cs-books@wiley.co.uk
      Visit our Home Page on http://eu.wiley.com

All Rights Reserved. No part of this book may be reproduced, stored in a retrieval
system or transmitted in any form or by any means, electronic, mechanical, photocopying,
recording, scanning or otherwise, except under the terms of the Copyright, Designs and
Patents Act 1988 or under the terms of a licence issued by the Copyright Licensing Agency Ltd,
90 Tottenham Court Road, London W1T 4LP, UK, without the permission in writing
of the Publisher. Requests to the Publisher should be addressed to the Permissions Department,
John Wiley & Sons Ltd, The Atrium, Southern Gate, Chichester, West Sussex PO19 8SQ,
England, or emailed to permreq@wiley.co.uk, or faxed to (+44) 1243 770620.

This publication is designed to provide accurate and authoritative information in regard to
the subject matter covered. It is sold on the understanding that the Publisher is not engaged
in rendering professional services. If professional advice or other expert assistance is
required, the services of a competent professional should be sought.

Other Wiley Editorial Offices

John Wiley & Sons Inc., 111 River Street, Hoboken, NJ 07030, USA

Jossey-Bass, 989 Market Street, San Francisco, CA 94103-1741, USA

Wiley-VCH Verlag GmbH, Boschstr. 12, D-69469 Weinheim, Germany

John Wiley & Sons Australia Ltd, 33 Park Road, Milton, Queensland 4064, Australia

John Wiley & Sons (Asia) Pte Ltd, 2 Clementi Loop #02-01, Jin Xing Distripark, Singapore
129809

John Wiley & Sons Canada Ltd, 22 Worcester Road, Etobicoke, Ontario, Canada M9W 1L1

Wiley also publishes its books in a variety of electronic formats. Some content that appears
in print may not be available in electronic books.

Novartis Foundation Symposium 278
viii + 232 pages, 20 figures, 1 tables

British Library Cataloguing in Publication Data

A catalogue record for this book is available from the British Library

ISBN 978-0-470-02626-7
ISBN 0-470-02626-X

Typeset in $10\frac{1}{2}$ on $12\frac{1}{2}$ pt Garamond by SNP Best-set Typesetter Ltd., Hong Kong.
Printed and bound in Great Britain by T. J. International Ltd, Padstow, Cornwall.
This book is printed on acid-free paper responsibly manufactured from sustainable forestry,
in which at least two trees are planted for each one used for paper production.

Contents

Participants

Ralph Adolphs   Room 331b, HSS 228-77, Caltech, Pasadena, CA 91125, USA

James Blair   NIMH Mood and Anxiety Disorders Programme, National Institutes of Health (NIH), 9000 Rockville Pike, Bethesda, MD 20892, USA

Sarah-Jayne Blakemore   Institute of Cognitive Neuroscience, University College London, Alexandra House, 17 Queen Square, London WC1N 3AR, UK

Sarah Brosnan   Emory University, Department of Anthropology, 1557 Pierce Drive, Atlanta, GA 30322, USA

Josep Call   Max Planck Institute for Evolutionary Anthropology, Deutscher Platz 6, D-04103 Leipzig, Germany

Frédérique de Vignemont   CNRS Institut des sciences cognitives, 67, Boulevard Pinel, F-69675 Bron cedex, France

Emmanuel Dupoux   École des Hautes Etudes en Sciences Sociales, Laboratoire de Science Cognitive et Psycholinguistique, 54 Boulevard Raspail, F-75270 Paris cedex 06, France

Robert Frank   327 Sage Hall, Johnson Graduate School of Management, Cornell University, Ithaca, NY 14853-6201, USA

Chris Frith   (*Chair*) Wellcome Department of Imaging Neuroscience, Institute of Neurology, University College London, 12 Queen Square, London WC1N 3BG, UK

Uta Frith   Institute of Cognitive Neuroscience & Department of Psychology, University College London, Alexandra House, 17 Queen Square, London WC1N 3AR, UK

Vittorio Gallese   Department of Neurosciences, Section of Physiology, Universita degli Studi Di Parma, Via Volturno 39, I-43100 Parma, Italy

Gyorgy Gergely   Institute for Psychological Research, Hungarian Academy of Sciences, P.O. Box 398, Budapest, H-1394, Hungary

Marc Hauser   Department of Psychology, Organismic & Evolutionary Biology, and Biological Anthropology, 33 Kirkland Street, Harvard University, Cambridge, MA 02138, USA

C. Neil Macrae   School of Psychology, University of Aberdeen, King's College, Aberdeen AB24 2UB, UK

Jorge Moll   Cognitive Neuroscience Section, National Institute of Neurological Disorders and Stroke, Building 10, Room 5C206, Bethesda, MD 20892-1440, USA

P. Read Montague   Department of Neuroscience, Baylor College of Medicine, Vivian Smith Building, Room S603, One Baylor Plaza, Houston, TX 77030, USA

Marian Sigman   Department of Psychology, UCLA, 1285 Franz Hall, Box 951563, Los Angeles, CA 90095-1563, USA

Joan B. Silk   UCLA Department of Anthropology, 341 Haines Hall, Box 951553, Los Angeles, CA 90095-1553, USA

Tania Singer   Wellcome Department of Imaging Neuroscience & Institute of Cognitive Neuroscience, University College London, Alexandra House, 17 Queen Square, London WC1N 3AR, UK

Tracy Spinrad   Department of Family and Human Development, Arizona State University, Tempe, AZ 85287-2502, USA

Paul A. M. Van Lange   Free University of Amsterdam, Department of Social Psychology, Van der Boechorststraat 1, Room 1B-41, 1081 BT Amsterdam, The Netherlands

Jonathan Wolff   Department of Philosophy, University College London, Gower Street, London WC1E 6BT, UK

Felix Warneken   Max Planck Institute for Evolutionary Anthropology, Department of Developmental and Comparative Psychology, Deutscher Platz 6, D-04103 Leipzig, Germany

Chair's introduction

Chris Frith

Wellcome Department of Imaging Neuroscience, Institute of Neurology, University College London, 12 Queen Square, London WC1N 3BG, UK

We're here to discuss empathy and fairness. In the last few years there have been dramatic changes in our attitude to concepts such as these. While we have always known that empathy and fairness describe a vital part of human culture, very few have had the courage to apply science to these topics. Now this has changed and there is much current research including computational models of fairness and brain imaging studies on the neural basis of empathy. One of the purposes of this meeting is to bring together people who have been studying these topics for some time with those of us who are completely new to the area. We have a lot to learn from each other.

This book contains contributions from people from many different disciplines, who have different approaches to this topic. We have neurophysiologists, psychologists, philosophers and economists, all asking different empirical questions about empathy and fairness. How do these processes evolve? How do they develop during the lifespan? How do they change as a result of damage to the brain? Given all these different approaches, I think the first thing we will discover is that we have different definitions of what empathy and fairness are. For example, at one extreme, empathy can refer to a form of automatic emotional contagion. At the other, it necessarily involves the action taken to reduce another's suffering. By the end of the meeting I hope we'll appreciate these differences and have a better understanding of how the evidence from our widely ranging studies could be made to fit together.

One obvious question is why have we put together empathy and fairness? In neuroscience there is not much overlap in the literature on these topics. Fairness tends to be studied within the realm of neuroeconomics, whereas empathy springs from the burgeoning studies that followed the discovery of mirror neurons. However, the two concepts are linked when we think of a possible basis for morality. We don't like to be treated unfairly ourselves and we empathise with others who are treated unfairly. We will act to correct unfairness and to prevent it recurring.

Furthermore, studying empathy and fairness will help us understand what emotions are for. In the past neuroscientists and experimental psychologists have taken a very British attitude to emotions: that is to say, we prefer not to have them and we are certainly not going to talk about them! This attitude can no longer be maintained in the face of all the evidence that emotions are not the enemy of decision making. Rather, they are crucial for making good decisions. One example I particularly like, which comes from economics, is the idea of anticipated regret. It helps us to make good decisions. People with orbitofrontal lesions can no longer represent anticipated regret (Camille et al 2004) and are well known to make very bad decisions.

Empathy and a sense of fairness are closely linked to emotions, and they play a key role in social interactions and social decision making. Our interactions are conducted so as to maximize fairness; on the other hand, the feeling of unfairness is a signal that something has to be done to change a situation. The sense of fairness is therefore part of a homeostatic mechanism which maintains the social status quo. I am very much influenced here by Bud Craig's suggestion that pain, like other emotions, is also part of a homeostatic mechanism: it is a signal that something must be done in order to reduce the pain or avoid it in the future (Craig 2003). Empathy for pain has the same role in a social interaction, acting as a signal that we must take action to reduce the pain of another. The feeling that someone else is being treated unfairly is a form of empathy which may well have the same neural signature as empathy for physical pain.

In terms of this homeostatic model it turns out that we British were right all along: in the ideal state, emotion is minimized. I am looking forward to calm and orderly interactions over the next few days.

References

Camille N, Coricelli G, Sallet J, Pradat-Diehl P, Duhamel JR, Sirigu A 2004 The involvement of the orbitofrontal cortex in the experience of regret. Science 304:1167–1170
Craig AD 2003 A new view of pain as a homeostatic emotion. Trends Neurosci 26:303–307

Embodied simulation: from mirror neuron systems to interpersonal relations

Vittorio Gallese

Dipartimento di Neuroscienze, Università di Parma, Via Volturno 39, 43100 Parma, Italy

Abstract. A direct form of 'experiential understanding' of others is achieved by modelling their behaviours as intentional experiences on the basis of the equivalence between what the others do and feel and what we do and feel. This modelling mechanism is embodied simulation. By means of embodied simulation we do not just 'see' an action, an emotion, or a sensation. Side by side with the sensory description of the observed social stimuli, internal representations of the body states associated with actions, emotions, and sensations are evoked in the observer, as if he/she would be doing a similar action or experiencing a similar emotion or sensation. Mirror neurons are likely the neural correlate of this mechanism. The mirror neuron matching systems map the different intentional relations in a compressed fashion, which is neutral about the specific quality or identity of the agentive/subjective parameter. By means of a shared neural state realized in two different bodies that nevertheless obey to the same functional rules, the 'objectual other' becomes 'another self'.

2006 Empathy and Fairness. Wiley, Chichester (Novartis Foundation Symposium 278) p 3–19

During the last decades, developmental psychology research has provided one of the major contributions to a new understanding of human social cognition. In the course of infancy and childhood, we all heavily rely on interactions with our caregivers and with other individuals to learn how to cope with the world. Developmental psychology, by providing an enormous amount of data, has literally revolutionized our way of looking at newborns and infants as cognitive agents. These results have shown, among other things, that at the very beginning of our life we almost immediately interact with others by *reproducing* some of their behaviours.

Several studies have shown that the capacity of infants to establish relations with 'others' is accompanied by the registration of behavioural invariance. As pointed out by Stern (1985), this invariance encompasses unity of locus, coherence of motion and coherence of temporal structure. This experience-driven process of constant remodelling is one of the building blocks of cognitive development, and it capitalizes upon coherence, regularity and predictability. Social identity guarantees all these features, henceforth its high social adaptive value. The experience of identity between infant and caregiver is *the* starting point for the development of social cognition.

The seminal study of Meltzoff & Moore (1977) and the subsequent research field it opened showed that newborns as young as 18 hours are capable of reproducing mouth and face movements displayed by the adult they are facing. That particular part of their body replies, though not in a reflex way, to movements displayed by the equivalent body part of someone else. More precisely, this means that newborns set into motion a part of their body they have no visual access to, but which nevertheless matches an observed behaviour. To put it crudely, visual information is transformed into motor information. The issue then consists in clarifying the nature of this peculiar feature and the possible underlying mechanisms. The relational character intrinsic to the interaction between any biological system and its environment appears to be a good candidate. Our environment is composed of a variety of lifeless forms of matter, and of a variety of 'alive stuff', whose peculiar character is more and more focused by the infant's immature eye. Individuals confront themselves with all possible kinds of 'external' objects, in virtue of their peculiar status of biological systems, thus by definition constrained in their peculiar 'modes of interaction' (see Gallese 2003).

Interpersonal relations are established at the very onset of our life, when a full-blown self-conscious subject of experience is not yet constituted. Yet, the absence of a subject doesn't preclude the presence of a primitive 'we-centric space', a paradoxical form of intersubjectivity without subject. The infant shares this space with others. The physical space occupied by the bodies of the adult-others is 'hooked up' to the body of the infant to compose a blended shared space. In a way, it is as if the mother, who creates and holds the fetus within her body during pregnancy, continues to hold and create the child in his/her first months and years of life, being both biologically and culturally connected in fundamental ways. This intersubjective process continues for the entire lifespan, becoming much richer and multifaceted, due to the wider range and meaning of interpersonal relations in the course of development.

The shared we-centric space enables the social bootstrapping of cognitive and affective development because it provides a powerful tool to detect and incorporate coherence, regularity and predictability in the course of the interactions of the individual with the environment. The we-centric space is paralleled by the development of perspectival spaces defined by the establishment of the capacity to distinguish self from other, as long as self-control develops. Within each of these newly acquired perspectival spaces information can be better segregated in discrete channels (visual, somatosensory, etc.) making the perception of the world more finely grained. The concurrent development of language contributes to further segregation from the original multimodal perceptive world, single characters or modalities of experience. Yet, the more mature capacity to segregate the modes of interaction, together with the capacity of carving out the subject and the object of the interaction, do not annihilate the shared we-centric space.

The shared intersubjective we-centric space progressively acquires a different role. It provides the self with the capacity to simultaneously entertain self-other identity and difference. Once the crucial bonds with the world of others are established, this space carries over to the adult conceptual faculty of socially mapping sameness and difference ('I am a different subject'). Within intersubjective relations, the other is a living oxymoron, being just a different self. Social identity, the 'selfness' we readily attribute to others, the inner feeling of 'being-like-you' triggered by our encounter with others, are the result of the preserved shared we-centric space. Self-other physical and epistemic interactions are shaped and conditioned by the same body and environmental constraints. This common relational character is underpinned, at the level of the brain, by neural networks that compress the 'who-done-it', 'who-is-it' specifications, and realize a narrower content state, a content that specifies what kinds of interaction or state are at stake. This narrower content is shared not only because of the shareable character of experience, but also because it is underpinned by shared neural mechanisms.

The posited important role of identity relations in constraining the cognitive development of our mind provides a strong motivation to investigate from a neuroscientific perspective the functional mechanisms, and their neural underpinnings, at the basis of the self-other identity. This will be the focus of the next sections.

The mirror neuron system for actions in monkeys and humans: empirical evidence

About 10 years ago a new class of premotor neurons was discovered in the ventral premotor cortex of the macaque monkey brain. These neurons discharge not only when the monkey executes goal-related hand actions like grasping objects, but also when observing other individuals (monkeys or humans) executing similar actions. They were called 'mirror neurons'[1] (Gallese et al 1996, Rizzolatti et al

---

[1] This paper is exclusively focused on the relationships among the mirror neuron system, embodied simulation and the experiential aspects of intersubjectivity. For sake of concision, many other issues related to mirror neurons and simulation will not be addressed here. The vast literature on the mirror neuron system in humans and its relevance for theory of mind, imitation and the evolution of language is reviewed and discussed in several papers (Gallese & Goldman 1998, Rizzolatti & Arbib 1998, Gallese 2003, Rizzolatti & Craighero 2004, Gallese et al 2004). For the analysis of the role played by embodied simulation in conceptual structure and content, see Gallese & Lakoff (2005).

1996). Neurons with similar properties were later discovered in a sector of the posterior parietal cortex reciprocally connected with area F5 (PF/PG mirror neurons; see Gallese et al 2002, Rizzolatti & Craighero 2004, Fogassi et al 2005).

Action observation causes in the observer the automatic activation of the same neural mechanism triggered by action execution. It has been proposed that this mechanism could be at the basis of a direct form of action understanding (Gallese et al 1996, 2004, Rizzolatti et al 2001).

Further studies carried out by our research group at the Department of Neuroscience of the University of Parma corroborated and extended the original hypothesis. It was shown that F5 mirror neurons are also activated when the final critical part of the observed action, that is, the hand–object interaction, is hidden (Umiltà et al 2001). A second study showed that a particular class of F5 mirror neurons, 'audiovisual mirror neurons', can be driven not only by action execution and observation, but also by the sound produced by the same action (Kohler et al 2002).

More recently, the most lateral part of area F5 was explored where a population of mirror neurons related to the execution/observation of mouth actions was described (Ferrari et al 2003). The majority of these neurons discharge when the monkey executes and observes transitive, object-related ingestive actions, such as grasping, biting or licking. However, a small percentage of mouth-related mirror neurons discharge during the observation of intransitive, communicative facial actions performed by the experimenter in front of the monkey ('communicative mirror neurons'; Ferrari et al 2003). Thus, mirror neurons seem also to underpin aspects of monkeys' social facial communication.

Several studies using different experimental methodologies and techniques have demonstrated also in the human brain the existence of a mirror neuron system matching action perception and execution. During action observation there is a strong activation of premotor and parietal areas, the likely human homologue of the monkey areas in which mirror neurons were originally described (for review, see Rizzolatti et al 2001, Rizzolatti & Craighero 2004, Gallese et al 2004). Furthermore, the mirror neuron matching system for actions in humans is somatotopically organized, with distinct cortical regions within the premotor and posterior parietal cortices being activated by the observation/execution of mouth-, hand- and foot-related actions (Buccino et al 2001).

The involvement of the motor system during observation of communicative mouth actions is also testified by the results of recent functional magnetic resonance imaging (fMRI) and transcranial magnetic stimulation (TMS) studies (Buccino et al 2004, Watkins et al 2003). The observation of communicative, or speech-related mouth actions, facilitate the excitability of the motor system involved in the production of the same actions.

Mirror neurons and the understanding of intentions

When an individual starts a movement aimed to attain a goal, such as picking up a pen, he/she has clear in mind what he/she is going to do, for example writing a note on a piece of paper. In this simple sequence of motor acts the final goal of the whole action is present in the agent's mind and is somehow reflected in each motor act of the sequence. The action intention, therefore, is set before the beginning of the movements. This also means that when we are going to execute a given action we can also predict its consequences.

Monkeys may exploit the mirror neuron system to optimize their social interactions. My hypothesis is that monkeys might entertain a rudimentary form of 'teleological stance', a likely precursor of a full-blown intentional stance. This hypothesis extends to the phylogenetic domain, the ontogenetic scenario proposed by Gergely & Csibra (2003) for human infants. New experiments are being designed in my lab to test this hypothesis.

But monkeys certainly do not entertain full-blown mentalization. Thus, what makes humans different? At present we can only make hypotheses about the relevant neural mechanisms underpinning the mentalizing abilities of humans, still poorly understood from a functional point of view. In particular, we do not have a clear neuroscientific model of how humans can understand the intentions promoting the actions of others they observe.

A given action can be originated by very different intentions. Suppose one sees someone else grasping a cup. Mirror neurons for grasping will most likely be activated in the observer's brain. A simple motor equivalence between the observed action and its motor representation in the observer's brain, however, can only tell us what the action is (it's a grasp) and not why the action occurred. Determining why action A (grasping the cup) was executed, that is, determining its intention, can be equivalent to detecting the goal of the still not executed and impending subsequent action B (say, drink from the cup).

In an fMRI study we recently published (Iacoboni et al 2005), participants watched three kinds of stimuli: grasping hand actions without a context, context only (a scene containing objects), and grasping hand actions embedded in contexts. In the latter condition the context suggested the intention associated with the grasping action (either drinking or cleaning up). Actions embedded in contexts, compared with the other two conditions, yielded a significant signal increase in the posterior part of the inferior frontal gyrus and the adjacent sector of the ventral premotor cortex where hand actions are represented. Thus, premotor mirror areas—areas active during the execution and the observation of an action—previously thought to be involved only in action recognition are actually also involved in understanding the 'why' of action, that is, the intention promoting it. Detecting the intention of Action A is equivalent to predicting its distal goal, that is, the goal of the subsequent Action B.

Similar findings were recently obtained in monkeys. Fogassi et al (2005) described a class of parietal mirror neurons whose discharge during the observation of an act (e.g. grasping an object), is conditioned by the type of not yet observed subsequent act (e.g. bringing the object to the mouth) specifying the overall action intention. Thus, these neurons not only code the observed motor act but also seem to allow the observing monkey to predict the agent's next action, henceforth his/her overall intention. It is possible to interpret this mechanism as the neural correlate of the dawning of more sophisticated mentalizing abilities, as those characterizing our species.

The statistical detection of which actions most frequently follow other actions, as they are habitually performed or observed in the social environment, can constrain preferential paths of inferences/predictions. It can be hypothesized that this can be accomplished by chaining different populations of mirror neurons coding not only the observed motor act, but also those that in a given context would normally follow. Ascribing intentions would therefore consist in predicting a forthcoming new goal. If this is true, it follows that one important difference between humans and monkeys could be the level of recursivity attained by the mirror neuron system in our species. According to this perspective, action prediction and the ascription of intentions are related phenomena, underpinned by the same functional mechanism. In contrast with what mainstream cognitive science would maintain, action prediction and the ascription of intentions—at least of simple intentions—do not appear to belong to different cognitive realms, but both pertain to embodied simulation mechanisms underpinned by the activation of chains of logically related mirror neurons (see Iacoboni et al 2005, Fogassi et al 2005).

Mirroring emotions and sensations

Emotions constitute one of the earliest ways available to the individual to acquire knowledge about its situation, thus enabling a reorganization of this knowledge on the basis of the outcome of the relations entertained with others. The coordinated activity of sensory–motor and affective neural systems results in the simplification and automatization of the behavioural responses that living organisms are supposed to produce in order to survive. The integrity of the sensory–motor system indeed appears to be critical for the recognition of emotions displayed by others (see Adolphs 2003), because the sensory–motor system appears to support the reconstruction of what it would feel like to be in a particular emotion, by means of simulation of the related body state. The implication of this process for empathy should be obvious.

A recently published fMRI study showed that experiencing disgust and witnessing the same emotion expressed by the facial mimicry of someone else, both activate the same neural structure—the anterior insula—at the same location (Wicker et al 2003). This shows that when we see the facial expression of someone else, and this perception leads us to experience a particular affective state, the other's emotion is constituted, experienced and therefore directly understood by means of an embodied simulation producing a shared body state. It is the activation of a neural mechanism shared by the observer and the observed to enable direct experiential understanding. A similar simulation-based mechanism has been proposed by Goldman & Sripada (2005) as 'unmediated resonance'.

Let us now examine somatic sensations as the target of our social perception. As repeatedly emphasized by phenomenology, touch has a privileged status in making possible the social attribution of lived personhood to others. 'Let's be in touch' is a common clause in everyday language, which metaphorically describes the wish of being related, being in contact with someone else. Such examples show how the tactile dimension can be intimately related to the interpersonal dimension.

New empirical evidence suggests that the first-person experience of being touched on one's body activates the same neural networks activated by observing the body of someone else being touched (Keysers et al 2004, Blakemore et al 2005). This double pattern of activation of the same somatosensory-related brain regions suggests that our capacity to experience and directly understand the tactile experience of others could be mediated by embodied simulation, that is, by the externally triggered activation of *some* of the same neural networks underpinning our own tactile sensations. A similar mechanism likely underpins our experience of the painful sensations of others (see Hutchison et al 1999, Singer et al 2004, Avenanti et al 2005).

Intentional attunement, embodied simulation and empathy

Various mirror neurons matching systems mediate between the multimodal experiential knowledge we hold of our lived body, and the experience we make of others. Such body-related experiential knowledge enables a direct grasping of the sense of the actions performed by others, and of the emotions and sensations they experience. Our capacity to conceive of the acting bodies of others as *persons* like us depends on the constitution of a shared meaningful interpersonal space. This 'shared manifold' (see Gallese 2001, 2003, 2005) can be characterized at the functional level as embodied simulation, a specific mechanism constituting a basic functional feature by means of which our brain/body system models its interactions with the world. Embodied simulation constitutes a crucial functional mechanism in social cognition, and it can be neurobiologically characterized. The different mirror neuron systems represent the sub-personal instantiation of embodied simulation.

When we confront the intentional behaviour of others, embodied simulation generates a specific phenomenal state of 'intentional attunement'. This phenomenal state in turn generates a peculiar quality of familiarity with other individuals, produced by the collapse of the others' intentions into the observer's ones. By means of embodied simulation we do not just 'see' an action, an emotion, or a sensation. Side by side with the sensory description of the observed social stimuli, internal representations of the body states associated with these actions, emotions, and sensations are evoked in the observer, 'as if' he/she would be doing a similar action or experiencing a similar emotion or sensation.

Any intentional relation can be mapped as a relation between a subject and an object. The mirror neuron matching systems described in this paper map the different intentional relations in a fashion that is neutral about the specific quality or identity of the agentive/subjective parameter. By means of a shared functional state realized in two different bodies that nevertheless obey to same functional rules, the 'objectual other' becomes 'another self'.

Of course, embodied simulation is not the only functional mechanism underpinning social cognition. The same actions performed by others in different contexts can lead the observer to radically different interpretations. Social stimuli can also be understood on the basis of the explicit cognitive elaboration of their contextual perceptual features, by exploiting previously acquired knowledge about relevant aspects of the situation to be analysed. Our capacity of attributing false beliefs to others, our most sophisticated mind reading abilities, likely involve the activation of large regions of our brain, certainly larger than a putative and domain-specific theory of mind module. Embodied simulation and the still poorly understood more sophisticated mentalizing cognitive skills, however, are not mutually exclusive. Embodied simulation, probably the most ancient mechanism from an evolutionary point of view, is experience-based, while the second mechanism can be characterized as a 'detached' cognitive description of an external state of affairs. It might well be the case that embodied simulation scaffolds the propositional, language-mediated mechanism. When the former mechanism is not present or malfunctioning, as perhaps in the autistic spectrum disorder (ASD), the latter can provide only a pale, detached account of the social experiences of others (see Gallese et al 2004). Recent evidence seems to support the hypothesis of ASD as at least in part due to a defective embodied stimulation (see Oberman et al 2005, Theoret et al 2005).

Conclusions

Social cognition is not only thinking about the contents of someone else's mind. Our brains, and those of other primates, have developed a basic functional mechanism, embodied simulation, which gives us an experiential insight of other minds. The neuroscientific evidence here reviewed suggests that social cognition is tractable at the neural level of description. This level is implicit, though, when the organism is confronting the intentional behaviour of others, it produces a specific phenomenal state of 'intentional attunement'. This phenomenal state generates a peculiar quality of familiarity with other individuals, produced by the collapse of the others' intentions into the observer's ones. This seems to be one important component of what being empathic is about.

However, self-other identity is not all there is in empathy. Empathy, in contrast to emotional contagion, entails the capacity to experience what others do experience, while being able to attribute these shared experiences to *others* and not to the self. The quality of our *erlebnis* of the external world and its content are constrained by the presence of other subjects that are intelligible, while preserving their alterity character. An alterity that is present also at the sub-personal level, instantiated by the different neural networks coming into play and/or by their different degree of activation when *I* act with respect to when others act, or when *I* experience an emotion or a sensation with respect to when others do the same.

References

Adolphs R 2003 Cognitive neuroscience of human social behaviour. Nat Rev Neurosci 4: 165–178

Avenanti A, Bueti D, Galati G, Aglioti SM 2005 Transcranial magnetic stimulation highlights the sensorimotor side of empathy for pain. Nat Neurosci 8:955–960

Blakemore S-J, Bristow D, Bird G, Frith C, Ward J 2005 Somatosensory activations during the observation of touch and a case of vision–touch synaesthesia. Brain 128:1571–1583

Buccino G, Binkofski F, Fink GR et al 2001 Action observation activates premotor and parietal areas in a somatotopic manner: an fMRI study. Eur J Neurosci 13:400–404

Buccino G, Lui F, Canessa N et al 2004 Neural circuits involved in the recognition of actions performed by nonconspecifics: An fMRI study. J Cogn Neurosci 16:114–126

Ferrari PF, Gallese V, Rizzolatti G, Fogassi L 2003 Mirror neurons responding to the observation of ingestive and communicative mouth actions in the monkey ventral premotor cortex. Eur J Neurosci 17:1703–1714

Fogassi L, Ferrari PF, Gesierich B, Rozzi S, Chersi F, Rizzolatti G 2005 Parietal lobe: From action organization to intention understanding. Science 302:662–667

Gallese V 2001 The 'shared manifold' hypothesis: from mirror neurons to empathy. J Consciousness Stud 8:33–50

Gallese V 2003 The manifold nature of interpersonal relations: The quest for a common mechanism. Phil Trans Royal Soc London B 358:517–528

Gallese V 2005 Embodied simulation: from neurons to phenomenal experience. Phenomenology Cog Sci 4:23–48

Gallese V, Goldman A 1998 Mirror neurons and the simulation theory of mind-reading. Trends Cogn Sci 12:493–501

Gallese V, Lakoff G 2005 The brain's concepts: The role of the sensory-motor system in reason and language. Cogn Neuropsychol 22:455–479

Gallese V, Fadiga L, Fogassi L, Rizzolatti G 1996 Action recognition in the premotor cortex. Brain 119:593–609

Gallese V, Fogassi L, Fadiga L, Rizzolatti G 2002 Action representation and the inferior parietal lobule. In Prinz W, Hommel B (eds) Attention and performance XIX. Oxford University Press, Oxford, p 247–266

Gallese V, Keysers C, Rizzolatti G 2004 A unifying view of the basis of social cognition. Trends Cogn Sci 8:396–403

Gergely G, Csibra G 2003 Teleological reasoning in infancy: the naive theory of rational action. TICS 7:287–292

Goldman A, Sripada CS 2005 Simulationist models of face-based emotion recognition. Cognition 94:193–213

Hutchison WD, Davis KD, Lozano AM, Tasker RR, Dostrovsky JO 1999 Pain related neurons in the human cingulate cortex. Nat Neurosci 2:403–405

Iacoboni M, Molnar-Szakacs I, Gallese V, Buccino G, Mazziotta J, Rizzolatti G 2005 Grasping the intentions of others with one's own mirror neuron system. PLOS Biol 3:529–535

Keysers C, Wickers B, Gazzola V, Anton J-L, Fogassi L, Gallese V 2004 A Touching sight: SII/PV activation during the observation and experience of touch. Neuron 42:335–346

Kohler E, Keysers C, Umiltà MA, Fogassi L, Gallese V, Rizzolatti G 2002 Hearing sounds, understanding actions: Action representation in mirror neurons. Science 297:846–848

Meltzoff AN, Moore MK 1977 Imitation of facial and manual gestures by human neonates. Science 198:75–78

Oberman LM, Hubbard EH, McCleery JP, Altschuler E, Ramachandran VS, Pineda JA 2005 EEG evidence for mirror neuron dysfunction in autism spectrum disorders. Cog Brain Res 24:190–198

Rizzolatti G, Arbib MA 1998 Language within our grasp. Trends Neurosci 21:188–194

Rizzolatti G, Craighero L 2004 The mirror neuron system. Ann Rev Neurosci 27: 169–192

Rizzolatti G, Fadiga L, Gallese V, Fogassi L 1996 Premotor cortex and the recognition of motor actions. Cog Brain Res 3:131–141

Rizzolatti G, Fogassi L, Gallese V 2001 Neurophysiological mechanisms underlying the understanding and imitation of action. Nat Rev Neurosci 2:661–670

Singer T, Seymour B, O'Doherty J, Kaube H, Dolan RJ, Frith CF 2004 Empathy for pain involves the affective but not the sensory components of pain. Science 303:1157–1162

Stern DN 1985 The interpersonal world of the infant. Karnac Books, London

Theoret H, Halligan E, Kobayashi M, Fregni F, Tager-Flusberg H, Pascual-Leone A 2005 Impaired motor facilitation during action observation in individuals with autism spectrum disorder. Curr Biology 15:84–85

Umiltà MA, Kohler E, Gallese V et al 2001 'I know what you are doing': a neurophysiological study. Neuron: 32:91–101

Watkins KE, Strafella AP, Paus T 2003 Seeing and hearing speech excites the motor system involved in speech production. Neuropsychologia 41:989–994

Wicker B, Keysers C, Plailly J, Royet J-P, Gallese V, Rizzolatti G 2003 Both of us disgusted in my insula: The common neural basis of seeing and feeling disgust. Neuron 40:655–664

DISCUSSION

C Frith: The key theme so far is the idea that we can actually share the experiences of other people because there are built-in brain mechanisms that somehow interpret what we see and recreate the experience in ourselves. Do people feel that this is sufficient to explain concepts such as empathy?

Singer: Clearly, this affect sharing mechanism is just one mechanism underlying what is broadly referred to as empathy. In addition to the ability to share other peoples' feelings, we also have to distinguish between self and other, and be able to modulate and control our empathic abilities. Thus, we do not always engage in empathy. Most of the time we actually do not empathize with others. Coming back to the shared affect mechanism or research on mirror neurons, I asked myself whether the emergence of such shared representations between self and other could not simply be accounted by associative learning mechanisms? Associative learning mechanisms could easily explain empathic responses in the action and the emotional domain. Do we need to implicate mirror neurons as a specific neuronal mechanism to account for the brain imaging data acquired? Could we not just assume that these are parts of an extended associative network connecting perceptual inputs to action or emotional outputs?

Gallese: Your question is about how this matching has been formed ontogenetically. This is an interesting point. Unfortunately, the truth is that we know very little about the ontogenetic aspects of mirror neurons. Colleagues of mine have started studying imitation in newborn monkeys, in collaboration with Steve Suomi. The results seem to suggest that macaque monkeys have early imitation, just as humans and chimps do. Some of these mechanisms could therefore be hard-wired. Nevertheless, there are other sets of data showing that the mirror matching system is highly plastic. For example, we now have data on two monkeys trained to grasp objects using a tool. In these monkeys mirror neurons also respond to the observation of tool use. This shows that by means of association the system can learn to respond to different stimuli. Why do you put associative and mirroring mechanisms as possibly conflicting? I don't understand this.

Singer: You are right. These accounts are not contradictory. One is the mechanism allowing these mirror neurons to emerge. The question is probably more related to how specific you assume mirror neurons to be. Do you assume that the mirror neurons you have measured in the monkey brain are very highly-specialized neurons, or just part of a huge network coding less specifically for all types of actions? I mean these neurons could be of a large associative network that has been formed by learned association by, for example, seeing yourself doing the hand action and thus associating the sight of a hand action to the motor performance of this action. The sight of a similar action in the other is then a cue to activate the network also containing the motor programme for this action.

Gallese: About one third of mirror neurons are highly specific. The remaining two thirds show a broader congruence between the executed and observed action. Self-observation coupled to action execution could indeed provide the starting association to be used to map the actions of others. The properties of mirror neurons are the outcome of the integrative work pooling together different input information.

Blair: Isn't the real issue the difference between the way that you describe the functional properties of mirror neurons for motor movements and the way that the concept is then translated with reference to empathy? Mirror neurons for motor movements cannot be established directly through simple association. To form an association between when you see someone else doing a movement and when you are seeing yourself doing the movement, a degree of translation is necessary. Whatever is going on, it has to be more complicated than what is going on in the pain studies. In a classic conditioning study you will see that some neurons in the amygdala will fire to pain and then come to fire to stimuli that actually anticipate the pain. You wouldn't want to call these neurons mirror neurons. There is a straight association process. If you have seen a stimulus approaching, your own hand anticipates pain, it is unsurprising from an association point of view that the same stimulus approaching another hand might lead to pain associated activity. This would occur on basic association grounds. This has to be a different computational process from that seen with mirror neurons.

Gallese: I'm happy to confine the tag 'mirror neuron' to motor-related aspects of inter-subjectivity. Nevertheless, I think I'm right in pooling together these different sets of empirical evidence, to the extent that they all point in the same direction. In order to make the content of my social perception meaningful this has to go through an activation of similar embodied mechanisms in my brain. If I want to understand how it feels to be disgusted or how it feel to be touched, this involves an activation of part of the brain that is actually activated when I am disgusted or touched. What binds together all the results I presented today is the underlying functional mechanism, what I qualify as embodied stimulation. It is a radically new perspective. Knowing 'how does it feel' is not the result of a hermeneutical process applied to sense data. This is certainly possible, but it is not what is likely to be going on in most of our daily social interactions.

Gergely: How do you account for the perception of Heiderian types of stimuli (Heider & Simmel 1944), and their intentional interpretation? These animated events involve 2D abstract figures such as circles and rectangles moving in relation to each other in ways that evoke strong intentional interpretations as goal-directed actions of interacting agents not only by adult perceivers but importantly by one-year-old infants as well (Gergely et al 1995, Gergely & Csibra 2003). However, the figures and their movements have no easy way of being directly mapped onto already existing motor representations of actions within the repertoire of the perceiver. This seems especially problematic when such events lack any movement cues suggesting animacy or agency (such as self-propulsion) but are still interpreted as goal-directed actions by 9- and 12-month-olds (Csibra et al 1999). To me this suggests that understanding and attributing goals to such perceived actions must be accomplished by some entirely different mechanism than the activation of corresponding motor action representations through some process of 'direct matching' or 'motor resonance' (see Csibra's recent arguments on this, Csibra, 2005.

Gallese: This may be true for the Heider and Simmel stimuli (Heider & Simmel 1944), but other abstract sequential stimuli have been used by R. Schubotz and colleagues. In that fMRI study they contrasted sequential biological actions and symbolic sequences of geometric shapes changing position on the screen. Subjects were required to predict whether the biological action or abstract sequence was goal directed or not. They had to anticipate the consequences of both abstract symbolic geometrical shape motion and biological motion. In both cases this led to strong activation of the ventral premotor cortex. Thus the abstract nature of stimuli doesn't prevent the involvement of the motor system. My bet is that we are going to learn more and more about the involvement of the sensory–motor system in the domain of syntax, for example. Embodied mechanisms may have something to say in this domain.

Gergely: If you get activation of the motor or mirror neuron system in such cases of non-biological motion of abstract figures that have no obvious similarity mapping on to the biomechanical motion properties of existing action schemes then I think you are postulating a rather mysterious mechanism of 'direct mapping' or 'motor resonance'. Without spelling out how you get from the perception of such abstract motion events to the activation of the premotor system, you have no viable model to account for the phenomena you are referring to.

Gallese: This is not necessarily due to the mirror system. When I am talking of premotor cortex, I am talking about of the neural correlates of different motor schemata.

Gergely: Doesn't this imply a kind of top–down route to activating the motor system? There has to be another system that infers and attributes the goal to the perceived action, which perhaps has a route of activating the motor system as a kind of action prediction or simulation mechanism.

Gallese: I know this line of argument. The problem is that no one knows this mysterious area where it is encoded. We stick to the extant empirical evidence and our claim is that we don't need to suppose an overarching top–down influence in order to have a neural mechanism that maps the goal. We already have it in the premotor system. We don't need to imply a further mechanism that maps the goal.

Gergely: I don't understand how the motor system becomes activated. What is the input that activates the motor system?

Gallese: This is what the motor system is there for: to guide actions by setting goals and end-states to be attained. The motor system is a lot more than a mere muscle controller! I should add that something we haven't looked for, but which must also play a key role, is the interaction between the reward system and the action system. Most likely we learn to code the fulfilment of a specific motor act as successfully leading to the acquisition of a target by means of a gating signal coming from reward-related brain areas. The interplay between the premotor cortex and reward-related areas is an interesting subject for future research.

Montague: I am missing something about where goals come from. Humans can and do establish top down goals. People routinely kill themselves for political protests. People can hold goals in mind for long periods. Surely you would say that there are goal-forming systems in the brain that would have access to these mirror systems.

Gallese: I am not denying this. My point is that you don't need to imply a top–down mechanism to explain *these* data. Certainly, we entertain the capacity to have a distal goal and pursue it. But in principle this does not necessarily imply that you need a radically different mechanism. It could only be a matter of adding power to the same basic architecture we have uncovered in the monkey.

Montague: It operates on low level things. When I come home at night and I am starving and I jam my hand into a bag of potato chips, right before it goes into my mouth my expanding waistline and declining dating life flash into my mind and make me stop. So you are restricting it to these classes of data, such as the impact of watching other people in pain. That is a complicated representation, to think of someone else having pain. I'd be hard-pressed to give a simple associative learning account of this. Even if a simple associative learning account could explain the data you presented, there is still one variable that is missing, which is that you have to assign it to someone else.

Singer: Exactly.

Montague: That itself is an abstract entity that is forming.

Gallese: My point is that having a mechanism that enables the sharing of a given content with someone else is the most critical aspect of the story. If you don't have this mechanism, you are not going anywhere. The self/other distinction in my opinion is not the most difficult problem in social cognition, neither from a theoretical, nor from an empirical point of view. The 'hard problem' in social cognition is to understand how the epistemic gulf separating single individuals can be overcome. The solipsistic attitude, inspired by folk psychology and purported by the approach of classic cognitive science, leaves this hard problem unsolved. The discovery of mirror neurons and related mirroring phenomena for the first time provides a neurophysiological mechanism that explains how the intersubjective epistemic gap can be filled.

Montague: Would it be fair to say that you see this as us coming pre-equipped with these rich processes of what it feels like for our own bodies to have experiences? I look and see you doing something, and the most efficient way for me to process this is to plug it back into the way I do the same thing. But not a lot has been done for super-ordinate goals with respect to the mirror systems.

Gallese: That is correct. We are at the beginning of this new research. Just give it time, I am confident that very soon we'll know a lot more also about superordinate goals.

Call: How do you go from here to prior goals, or predicting new instances of some behaviour?

Gallese: I find it more interesting to pursue a line of research that is trying to emphasize cognitive continuity rather than sudden jumps. To oversimplify the issue, a quantitative leap forward can buy you a qualitative leap forward. We don't need to think about new areas or new magic cells we have and monkeys don't. The level of recursivity attained by the human brain is one possible explanation for humans' much more sophisticated social skills. We can run all these simulations without being driven by the local context. I can close my eyes and think what I will be doing in two weeks' time. From a qualitative point of view, this doesn't seem to be dramatically different from what a monkey can do. Perhaps it is just the way our brains are wired that enables us to have this greater predictive capacity or ability to entertain distal goals well before their execution.

Call: In the experiment you mentioned with the monkeys, where grasping to eat or grasping to play took place, in that case the monkey has experienced both and eventually discriminates both.

Gallese: Yes, there is also contextual information that helps the monkey.

Hauser: I want to go back to your sense of continuity. I can see the excitement surrounding these imitation results, but of course they stand in contrast to 50 years of failure to show imitation in monkeys. The story that has come out from your group is that there is an almost seamless connection between the physiological recordings and what humans seem to do. Is this really how you see it? That there is no difference in the capacity to form intentions, create goals and experience empathy?

Gallese: There is a huge difference between the animal and human data.

Hauser: If you run a cognitive subtraction, what is different? The way you argued today, I don't hear a difference.

Gallese: The paper was meant to highlight the similarities, not focus on the differences.

Hauser: What is left? What gives us as humans a particular signature?

Gallese: I don't know. One possibility would be that these mechanisms can use much more computational power, plus the development of language which gives an incredible leap forward socially.

Hauser: For me, language is too much of a throwaway. Saying that language is involved doesn't explain what's going on, how language is involved or what aspect of language is doing the work. Let's go back to empathy. There is nothing in the animal literature that you have shown that has to do with emotion. You have the human studies which are claiming to be correlates of emotional experience, but there is nothing on the animal side. This is a big gap. Is there a case where an animal watches someone experience pain, for example?

Gallese: Colleagues of mine have started doing these sorts of experiments in the rat. The plan is to go soon into the monkey's insula.

Hauser: The simple experiment you could do, which would be ethical in monkeys, would be to use their vocalizations which are already coding information about emotion. The prediction is that when they produce a vocalization, hearing that call would be a trigger, and this would get around the association problem. It looks like the morphology of the signal is sometimes coded innately. I was intrigued that you were able to run such a natural experiment without any training at all. Now, if you can link the vocalization up to the emotions you have a natural experiment.

Gallese: We used chimpanzee vocalization as a stimulus to show the specificity of activation of audio–visual mirror neurons to the sounds produced by hand actions and it didn't work. But you are right, although it is really hard to induce a monkey to vocalize. You can record vocalizations and play them back to the monkey, but if you want to correlate the coding of the vocalization with the production, you also need to record the neuron when the monkey is actively producing the vocalization, which is a hell of a job.

Warneken: You said that this system creates an interpersonal space. If it is the case that an action is easier to understand when it is part of one's behavioural repertoire, it could also be that this goes beyond species barriers. Wouldn't this mandatory pre-rational process lead to false positives?

Gallese: This is what happens. I have friends literally in love with their pet boa constrictor!

Warneken: This means that there has to be another system coming in. What would that other system be? Is it something like face recognition?

Gallese: One thing that has been neglected so far is the specific quality of the observer. When we put people in the scanner we presume that our brains are wired up the same way. Personality traits can make a big difference. Our own social and cognitive history can make us react to the same stimulus in a different way. An encouraging line of research will be to show different patterns of activation induced by the same stimuli in subjects who have been screened before in a double blind way according to different personality trait ratings. I didn't include this in my paper. The take-home message of my short paper was that in order to start talking about empathy, we need a neural mechanism that enables us to bridge the gap.

De Vignemont: For philosophers mirror neurons are of great interest, because they could give a direct grasp on other people's feeling or thinking. However, in your account of intentions, you suggest that we have to *infer* the goal. Inferring is the opposite of a direct grasp. If we have indeed to infer the intention, then the mirror neurons account loses part of its interest. More specifically, in Fogassi et al (2005), monkeys have to put an apple into their mouth or on their shoulder. It would have been interesting to see what would happen if they had to put an inedible, neutral object in their mouth. Then one would really see whether they can detect intention, because the action would be exactly the same.

Gallese: This is what they did: they described this in the paper.

De Vignemont: The object was placed into a container located near the monkey's mouth, not in the mouth itself.

Gallese: It is a kind of statistical evaluation of the situation. Context, stimulus and action. Some kind of stimuli can make a given intention more predictable than others. Indeed, if the quality of the object that should induce that intention to be activated is patently falsified because the action is different, they saw some of the neurons decrease the discharge rate. In a sense it is a probabilistic mechanism. The mechanism couldn't possibly work without other brain regions that carry out this type of analysis of the quality of the object.

De Vignemont: Thus, we go back to the question whether mirror neurons by themselves suffice to provide a direct grasp of intentions. It rather seems that intention understanding relies partly on mirror neurons, partly on other brain areas. Mirror neurons are not sufficient. Understanding intentions requires inferring from the goal, from the context and from the movement. If this is really the case, then one cannot claim that we know the intentions of others in the same way that we know our own intentions through the mirror system. We have a direct knowledge of our intentions, while we have only an inferential indirect access to someone else's intentions. Mirror neurons cannot solve by themselves the problem of other minds.

Gallese: The interest of this approach is that it reduces the space to be investigated relative to the non-direct or top–down mechanisms. It may enable us to focus more specifically on the highly relevant top–down mechanism in social cognition by showing that a large part of the job is done at a lower level. This doesn't exclude higher-level mechanisms, but it enables us to focus our investigation.

References

Csibra G 2005 Mirror neurons or emulator neurons? http://mirrorneurons.free.fr/Cisbramirrorfunction.pdf

Csibra G, Gergely G, Biró S, Koós O, Brockbank M 1999 Goal-attribution and without agency cues: The perception of 'pure reason' in infancy. Cognition 72:237–267

Fogassi L, Ferrari PF, Gesierich B, Rozzi S, Chersi F, Rizzolatti G 2005 Parietal lobe: from action organization to intention understanding. Science 308:662–667

Gergely G, Csibra G 2003 Teleological reasoning about actions: the naïve theory of rational action. Trends Cog Sci 7:287–292

Gergely G, Nádasdy Y, Csibra G, Bíró S 1995 Taking the intentional stance at 12 months of age. Cognition 56:165–193

Heider F, Simmel M 1944 An experimental study of apparent behavior. Am J Psychol 57:243–259

The neuronal basis of empathy and fairness

Tania Singer[1]

Institute of Cognitive Neuroscience & Wellcome Department of Imaging Neuroscience, University College of London, WC1N 3AR London, UK

Abstract. The emerging fields of social neuroscience and neuroeconomics have started to investigate the neural foundations of empathy and fairness. Even though not frequently linked, both concepts point to humans as altruistic beings who care for others. Recently social neuroscientists have measured brain activity associated with different empathic processes and revealed common neural responses when feeling sensations such as disgust, touch or pain in ourselves, and when perceiving someone else being disgusted, touched or in pain. At the same time, research in neuroeconomics has used game theoretical paradigms to study our sense of fairness. Several functional magnetic resonance imaging (fMRI) studies show involvement of anterior insula and anterior cingulate cortex in response to unfair compared with fair offers during such monetary exchange games. Interestingly, the same brain regions are also involved in empathy for pain or disgust of others. More generally, anterior insula cortex is suggested to subserve neural representations of feeling and bodily states in the self and may play a crucial role for the emergence of social emotions related to others.

2006 Empathy and Fairness. Wiley, Chichester (Novartis Foundation Symposium 278) p 20–40

Empathy broadly refers to the process that allows us to feel for others, that is, to share the feelings and emotions of others. Humans can feel empathy for other people in a wide array of contexts: for basic emotions and sensations such as anger, fear, sadness, joy and pain as well as for more complex emotions such as guilt, embarrassment and love. It has been proposed that, for most people, empathy is the process that motivates prosocial behaviour and prevents us doing harm to others. An absence of empathy is what characterizes psychopaths who hurt others without feeling guilt or remorse (Blair 1995).

Although recent research on empathy seems to suggest that brain responses to other people's emotional responses are automatic, there are clearly circumstances under which we do not share the same feeling as others. Imagine, for example, that someone who does the same job as you is told that she will get twice your salary. The other person may be very happy with her extra salary, but you would not share this happiness as you would consider the situation unfair. This case

---

[1] Present address Center for Social Neuroscience and Neuroeconomics, University of Zurich, Blümlisalpstrasse 10, CH-8006 Zürich

illustrates the ubiquitous feeling of fairness and justice. The notion of fairness is not only crucial in interpersonal interaction with others (within the family, the workplace or with strangers) but also guides people's behaviour in impersonal economic and political domains.

Our sense of fairness has become the focus of many modern economic theories (e.g. Fehr & Schmidt 1999, 2003). In contrast to the prominent self-interest hypothesis of classic economics which assumes that all people are exclusively motivated by their self-interest, scholars have pointed out that human beings are also strongly motivated by other-regarding preferences such as the concern for fairness and reciprocity. Evolutionary anthropologists have also searched for evidence for prosocial behaviour in non-human species. Recently, Brosnan & deWaal (2003) found that capuchin monkeys react negatively, to the extent that they refuse to continue cooperating in an exchange game for food (cucumber), when they see another monkey receiving a better food reward (grape) for equal work. In contrast to these findings, however, Joan Silk and colleagues observed that chimpanzees do not show prosocial behavior when they were given the opportunity to actively provide benefits to others at no cost to themselves (Silk et al 2005). In this chapter I will provide a short overview of imaging research on empathy and fairness and will then discuss their possible links and differences.

The study of empathy

In the past few years, the study of the social and emotional brain has captured the interest of many researchers from a diverse range of disciplines. A new interdisciplinary field, *social cognitive neuroscience*, has emerged. There have been several special issues of science devoted to this topic and a number of review articles (e.g. Adolphs 2003, Ochsner & Lieberman 2001, Frith & Wolpert 2004).

The study of empathy has become the focus of recent investigation in social neuroscience and can be contrasted with research on a related topic, Theory of Mind (ToM). In contrast to ToM, which refers to the process of attributing propositional attitudes to another person (e.g. desires, beliefs and intentions), the ability to empathize refers to the process which allows us to experience what it feels like for another person to experience a certain emotion or sensation (e.g. qualia). The capacity to understand another person's emotions by sharing their affective states, such as sharing the grief of a close friend, is fundamentally different in nature from the capacity to understand their thoughts and intentions, the latter lacking a bodily sensation.

How can we understand what someone else feels when he or she experiences emotions or bodily sensations such as pain, touch or tickling, in the absence of any emotional or sensory stimulation to our own body? Influenced by perception–action models of motor behaviour and imitation (Prinz 1998), Preston & de Waal (2002) proposed a neuroscientific model of empathy, suggesting that observation or imagination of another person in a particular emotional state automatically activates a representation of that state in the observer with its associated autonomic and somatic responses. The term 'automatic' in this case refers to a process that does not require conscious and effortful processing but which can nevertheless be inhibited or controlled.

In the last three years, several imaging studies have revealed brain networks associated with different empathic responses in the domain of touch, smell and pain (Blakemore et al 2005, Jackson et al 2005, Keysers et al 2004, Morrison et al 2004, Singer et al 2004b, 2006, Wicker et al 2003). Wicker et al (2003) showed activity in the anterior insula (AI) and anterior cingulate cortex (ACC) both when experiencing disgust, and to the observation of another's disgusted facial expression. Accordingly, lesions of the insula result in impairment in experiencing disgust in the self, and in the recognition of disgust in others. (Calder 2000, Adolphs et al 2003). Similarly, two studies indicate the recruitment of somatosensory areas when volunteers were touched on different parts of their body, and when they watched someone else being touched in a video (Blakemore et al 2005, Keysers et al 2004).

Singer et al (2004b, 2006) expanded these approaches by measuring empathy for pain *in vivo* and identified both shared and unique networks involved in the vicarious experience of pain. To measure empathic responses *in vivo* she brought couples into the same scanner environment and compared the brain activity of the female partner while receiving painful stimulation of her own hand or watching cues indicating that her husband sitting next to the scanner was receiving painful stimulation. The results suggest that parts, but not the whole, of the 'pain matrix' were activated when empathizing with the pain of others. Activity in the primary and secondary somatosensory cortex/posterior insula contralateral to the stimulated hand was only observed when receiving pain (but see Avenanti et al 2005 and discussion of Singer & Frith 2005). In contrast, bilateral AI, the rostral ACC, brainstem, and cerebellum were activated when volunteers either received pain or a signal that a loved one was experiencing pain. These areas have been shown to be involved in the processing of the affective component of pain, that is, how unpleasant the pain feels. Interestingly, individual differences in empathy revealed by a standard empathy questionnaire were highly correlated with activity in these empathy-related areas. In summary, both the experience of pain to oneself and the knowledge that a loved-one is experiencing pain activates the same affective pain circuits. This suggests that we use representations of our own emotional response to pain in order to understand how the other feels when in pain.

The results of three recent independent studies indicate that empathic responses extend to unfamiliar people and that they are modulated by the affective link between people. Activity in ACC and AI has been also observed when volunteers watched still pictures depicting only body parts in painful situations (Jackson et al 2005) or videos showing a needle pricking the back of a hand (Morrison et al 2004). The findings of a recent study by Singer et al (2006) indicate that the magnitude of empathic responses in ACC and AI is modulated by the degree of familiarity between two persons and by whether the 'object of empathy' is liked or disliked. In this study actors pretended to be naïve volunteers participating with a real volunteer in two independent experiments; one on 'social exchange', the other on 'processing of pain'. In the first experiment, the two confederates repeatedly played a sequential Prisoner's Dilemma Game in the position of the second mover with the volunteer. One actor played fairly; they reciprocated cooperative moves by the volunteer with cooperative moves of their own; the other actor played unfairly and defected in response to cooperative moves by the volunteer. Post-experimental questionnaires showed that volunteers rated the fair actor to be a person they liked and found attractive and agreeable whereas the unfair actor was rated as unpleasant, dislikeable and unattractive. Moreover, most of the men (but not the women) indicated that they were angry with the unfair player, and they expressed the view that unfair player deserved to receive pain. These results are consistent with findings of a previous imaging study which revealed emotion-related brain activation in responses to faces of people who had previously cooperated or defected (Singer et al 2004a).

In the second part of the experiment, all three players participated in a pain study that expanded on the approach by Singer et al (2004b). One actor sat on each side of the scanner, enabling the scanned volunteer to observe coloured cues indicating high or low pain stimulation to their hand or to those of the fair or unfair players. Both men and women showed *increased* activation in ACC and AI when observing the unfamiliar but likeable person receiving painful stimulation. Interestingly, however, men but not women showed *reduced* activation in ACC and AI when they were informed that the player who previously played unfairly in the Prisoner's Dilemma game received painful shocks. Instead of empathy-related activity, men showed *enhanced* activity in the nucleus accumbens, an area known to play a key role in reward processing (e.g. O'Doherty 2004, Schultz 2000). Moreover, the magnitude of this reward-related activity increased with the strength of the subjectively expressed desire for revenge as elicited in post-scan questionnaires. These results suggest that both women and men show empathic responses towards unfamiliar people who had previously acted fairly, while men inhibit their empathic response towards an unfair player who they dislike. In fact, men seem to have engaged in reward-related processing—as indicated by the activation of the nucleus accumbens—when the unfair player received pain. This finding is in agreement with the results of a recent imaging study that reports similar reward-related activity when players could punish defectors in a sequential Prisoner's Dilemma game by delivering punishment points at personal costs (DeQuervain et al 2004). Further experiments are necessary to confirm the gender specificity of this effect; however, it could explain a predominant role of males in the maintenance of justice and punishment of norm violation in human societies.

The study of fairness

The study by Singer et al (2006) provides one example of how the concept of fairness and empathy can be combined within one study. In this study, however, playing fairly and unfairly was used to induce positive and negative emotions to assess any modulation of empathic brain responses. The focus was not on measuring brain responses underlying the processing of fair and unfair offers.

In the emerging field of neuroeconomics, however, the neural basis of fairness and social exchange has been directly explored by assessing brain activity of volunteers while playing versions of economic games developed in the framework of game theory such as the Prisoner's Dilemma Game, the Ultimatum Game or reciprocal trust games (e.g. Rilling et al 2002, Sanfey et al 2003, Singer et al 2004a). Sanfey et al, for example, scanned participants who responded to fair and unfair offers in an Ultimatum Game. Less fair offers activated the insula and the ACC bilaterally. Volunteers with stronger insula activation in response to unfair offers were also more likely to reject these offers. These data were not simply due to the receipt of less money because they were stronger when coming from human, as compared to computer, players.

In another study, Singer et al (2004a) assessed brain responses to faces of people who had been previously experienced as fair or unfair players through repeated play of a sequential Prisoners Dilemma game. To manipulate moral responsibility, players were either introduced as intentional or non-intentional agents. Perceiving faces of fair relative to neutral faces (players who have not been associated with either a fair or an unfair strategy), engendered increased activity in a brain network found to be relevant for the processing of socially salient stimuli (left amygdala, bilateral anterior insula, fusiform gyrus and posterior superior temporal sulcus [STS]). In addition, perceiving the face of a player who had intentionally compared to non-intentionally engaged in fair play elicited activity in reward-related areas (ventral striatum and lateral orbitofrontal cortex), a finding suggesting that fair play and social cooperation is inherently rewarding. These findings are supported by those of a study performed by Rilling and colleagues which showed that mutual cooperation while playing a simultaneous Prisoner's Dilemma game with another partner yielded stronger activation of brain reward-circuitry than mutual cooperation with a computer partner, even though the latter resulted in the same monetary payoffs (Rilling et al 2002).

King-Casas et al (2005) recently extended the former approaches using a similar repeated trust game as in the Singer et al study but now investigating the online dynamics of the expression and repayment of trust between two interacting brains with hyperscanning techniques. Consistent with previous studies, they also observed activity in the head of the caudate nucleus responding more strongly to benevolent than to malevolent reciprocity. Moreover, this study revealed that this region does not only compute information about the fairness of a social partner's decision but also about the intention to repay that decision with trust. Interestingly, similar to reward prediction errors in the animal literature, this signal moves forward in time as the second mover builds up a model about the first mover's reputation (King Casas et al 2005). In sum, these findings indicate that game theoretical paradigms provide powerful tools to investigate neural correlates of social cooperation, trust and its violation. The latter seems to be associated with emotion-related activity (AI, ACC); while positive reciprocation elicited activity in reward-related areas.

What do empathy and fairness have in common?

We can see from this brief review of the literature that empathy and fairness are both emerging topics in the new fields of social neuroscience and neuroeconomics. However, empathy and fairness, and their neural and psychological underpinnings, are rarely linked and discussed together even though they share common features. Both are social emotions arising only when embedded in the context of human interaction, and both point to the human being as altruistic, whether because he feels for the other or because he has a sense of social justice.

Another commonality seems to be that both empathy and fairness rely on rather automatic non-volitional processes. Without a great deal of thought, we quickly get a feeling of whether something is fair or unfair. When we see a loved-one crying we get tears in our eyes without having to engage in effortful cognitive reasoning processes. Note that in none of the studies on empathy and social exchange reviewed above were volunteers asked to give any explicit judgements about other people's feelings or the degree of perceived fairness. Volunteers were scanned while merely passively viewing others in pain, or receiving fair or unfair offers by other players. Note, however, that the results of the latest empathy study by Singer et al (2006) indicate that although empathic responses to pain seems to be elicited rather automatically they can nevertheless be modulated or even absent.

Future research will have to identify the brain mechanisms underlying the control of empathic responses and clarify the contextual factors modulating the presence and absence of empathic brain responses. Similarly, our sense of fairness is a complex multi-level construct and is probably also modulated by a variety of contextual and cognitive appraisal factors.

This literature review revealed another similarity: activity in the AI and ACC was enhanced when volunteers were empathizing with the pain or the disgust of others, and when volunteers were being treated unfairly during a monetary exchange game. What could the general underlying function of these regions be? We know that the insular cortex plays a crucial role in processing disgust, pain and other sensory qualities such as taste. The ACC has been ascribed a multitude of functions, including the processing of pain, arousal, cognitive conflict and emotion regulation.

More generally, it was suggested that these regions represent a crucial part of the human interoceptive cortex (Craig 2002) and subserve neural representations of internal bodily and feeling states (Critchley et al 2001, 2004, Damasio 1994). Bud Craig has developed a detailed model based on anatomical observations suggesting that an image of the body's internal state is first mapped to the brain by afferents that provide input to thalamic nuclei, sensorimotor cortices and posterior dorsal insula. In humans this modality-specific sensory representation of the physiological condition of the body in the posterior insula is initially re-represented in the AI on the same side of the brain, and then, by way of a callosal pathway, remapped to the other side of the brain in the right AI. Such a second-order re-representation in right AI is assumed to subserve subjective feelings and the awareness of a physical self as a feeling entity (see also Critchley et al 2001, Damasio 1994). At the same time, afferents also project by way of the medial dorsal thalamic nucleus to produce behavioural drive in ACC. Thus, direct activation of both the insula (limbic sensory cortex) and the ACC (the limbic motor cortex) may correspond to a simultaneous generation of both a feeling and an affective motivation with its attendant autonomic effects.

Indeed imaging studies focusing on the relationship between peripheral measures of arousal and brain activity give robust evidence for the crucial role of rostral ACC and AI cortices in the representation of internal bodily states of arousal as well as the awareness of these states (Critchley et al 2001, 2003, 2004). In a recent study Critchley demonstrated that activity and size of the right anterior insula was positively associated with the degree to which volunteers were aware of their own heartbeat (Critchley et al 2004).

Based on the findings of empathy-related activity in the AI, I suggest that this region may not only subserve representation of our own internal bodily and feeling states, but may also play a crucial role in the emergence of social emotions, that is the understanding of other people's emotions and their relation to ourselves (e.g. Singer et al 2004b). I further suggest that these cortical representations allow us to anticipate and predict affective outcomes of events for ourselves *and* for other people. Accordingly, these neural representations would allow future outcomes concerning the emotional world to be modelled and therefore predicted, even in the absence of any emotional stimulation to the self.

To explore these issues in more detail we are presently conducting a study investigating the combination of both concepts, namely empathic responses for fair and unfair dyadic interactions. In this study we are assessing brain responses in volunteers while they either receive monetary offers from other players (self condition) or watch another player receiving fair or unfair monetary offers while not being directly involved (empathy condition). To control for brain responses associated simply with gaining or loosing money, we have again included games in which volunteers play with freely intentional agents and players 'who have been told by a computer what to offer'.

The goal of this study is to identify common and unique brain networks recruited when we directly or vicariously experience fair and unfair offers. Furthermore, we aim to assess the degree to which empathizing motivates volunteers to engage in reward or punishment. We speculate that if volunteers empathize with the recipient of fair and unfair offers while watching two other people playing (third-party games), then these volunteers should also be motivated to reward and punish the person making the offer even though they have not personally been involved.

To assess whether there is evidence for altruistically motivated *third-party* punishment as well as altruistic reward volunteers were given the possibility to deliver punishment or reward points with a ratio of $1:3$, that is, 3% of the other player's total points were added (reward) or subtracted (punishment) while the volunteers had to endure a personal cost of 1% of their own total points.

As Fig. 1 illustrates, the results of a first pilot study including 16 women and 17 men revealed that both men and women were willing to reward and punish players who had cooperated or defected in previous interactions. Interestingly people were also willing to reward and punish others when they were not the recipient of the offer, but had instead observed the player make the offer to another player. As expected, the amount of reward and punishment in the empathy condition was significantly less than in the self condition. These findings suggest the involvement of empathic responses towards third parties. Further analysis of imaging data collected during this experiment will aim to determine whether similar brain networks (AI and ACC) are involved in the emotional responses to fairness violation in both self and others. The strength of these brain responses should be positively correlated with subjective fairness ratings and the amount of reward and punishment points delivered.

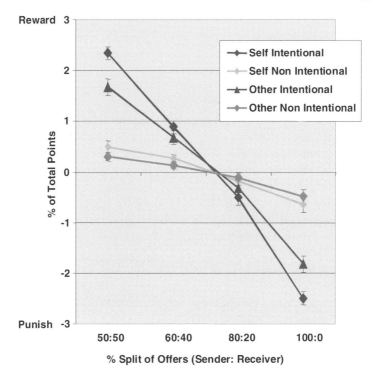

FIG. 1.   Altruistic punishment and reward for first-party and third-party games. The figure illustrates the average amount of reward and punishment points (in % of their total points) subjects are willing to invest to punish or reward players who had previously made fair or unfair monetary offers. Each % point invested results in three times % points of reward or punishment for the other. Average reward and punishment points are plotted as a function of the sender's previous offer ranging from 50:50 splits to 100:0 splits (the sender kept everything and offered nothing). The sender could either act intentionally (free to decide) or non-intentionally (told by a computer what to offer) and the subjects were either receiver of the offers (self) or only passively watching two other players exchanging offers (others).

References

Adolphs R 2003 Cognitive neuroscience of human social behaviour. Nat Rev Neurosci 4:
    165–178
Adolphs R, Tranel D, Damasio AR 2003 Dissociable neural systems for recognizing emotions.
    Brain Cogn 52:61–69
Avenanti A, Bueti D, Galati G, Aglioti SM 2005 Transcranial magnetic stimulation highlights
    the sensorimotor side of empathy for pain. Nat Neurosci 8:955–960
Blair RJR 1995 A cognitive developmental approach to morality: Investigating the psychopath.
    Cognition 57:1–29
Blakemore SJ, Bristow D, Bird G, Frith C, Ward J 2005 Somatosensory activations during the
    observation of touch and a case of vision-touch synaesthesia. Brain 128:1571–1583

Brosnan SF, De Waal FB 2003 Monkeys reject unequal pay. Nature 425:297–299
Calder AJ, Keane J, Manes F, Antoun N, Young AW 2000 Impaired recognition and experience of disgust following brain injury. Nat Neurosci 3:1077–1078
Craig AD 2002 How do you feel? Interoception: the sense of the physiological condition of the body. Nat Rev Neurosci 3:655–666
Critchley HD, Mathias CJ, Dolan RJ 2001 Neuroanatomical basis for first- and second-order representations of bodily states. Nat Neurosci 4:207–212
Critchley HD, Mathias CJ, Josephs O et al 2003 Human cingulate cortex and autonomic control: converging neuroimaging and clinical evidence. Brain 126:2139–2152
Critchley HD, Wiens S, Rotshtein P, Ohman A, Dolan RJ 2004 Neural systems supporting interoceptive awareness. Nat Neurosci 7:189–195
Damasio AR 1994 Descartes' Error. Putman, New York
de Quervain DJ, Fischbacher U, Treyer V et al 2004 The neural basis of altruistic punishment. Science 305:1254–1258
Fehr E, Schmidt KM 1999 A theory of fairness, competition, and cooperation. Quar J Econ 114:817–868
Fehr E, Schmidt KM 2003 Theories of fairness and reciprocity—evidence and economic applications. In: Dewatripont M, Hansen L, Turnovsky St (eds) Advances in economics and econometrics—8th World Congress, Econometric Society Monographs. Cambridge University Press, Cambridge, p 208–257
Frith C, Wolpert DM 2004 The neuroscience of social interaction: decoding, imitating, and influencing the actions of others. Oxford University Press, New York
Jackson PL, Meltzoff AN, Decety J 2005 How do we perceive the pain of others? A window into the neural processes involved in empathy. Neuroimage 24:771–779
Keysers C, Wicker B, Gazzola V, Anton JL, Fogassi L, Gallese V 2004 A touching sight: SII/PV activation during the observation and experience of touch. Neuron 42:335–346
King-Casas B, Tomlin D, Anen C, Camerer CF, Quartz SR, Montague PR 2005 Getting to know you: reputation and trust in a two-person economic exchange. Science 308:78–83
Morrison I, Lloyd D, di Pellegrino G, Roberts N 2004 Vicarious responses to pain in anterior cingulate cortex: is empathy a multisensory issue? Cogn Affect Behav Neurosci 4:270–278
O'Doherty JP 2004 Reward representations and reward-related learning in the human brain: insights from neuroimaging. Curr Opin Neurobiol 14:769–776
Ochsner KN, Lieberman MD 2001 The emergence of social cognitive neuroscience. Am Psychol 717–734
Preston SD, de-Waal FBM 2002 Empathy: Its ultimate and proximate bases. Behav Brain Sci 25:1–72
Prinz W 1997 Perception and action planning. Eur J Cogn Psychol 9:129–154
Rilling J, Gutman D, Zeh T, Pagnoni G, Berns G, Kilts C 2002 A neural basis for social cooperation. Neuron 35:395–405
Sanfey AG, Rilling JK, Aronson JA, Nystrom LE, Cohen JD 2003 The neural basis of economic decision-making in the Ultimatum Game. Science 300:1755–1758
Schultz W 2000 Multiple reward signals in the brain. Nat Rev Neurosci 1:199–207
Silk JB, Brosnan SF, Vonk J et al 2005 Chimpanzees are indifferent to the welfare of unrelated group members. Nature 437:1357–1359
Singer T, Frith C 2005 The painful side of empathy. Nat Neurosci 8:845–846
Singer T, Kiebel SJ, Winston JS, Dolan RJ, Frith CD 2004a Brain responses to the acquired moral status of faces. Neuron 41:653–662
Singer T, Seymour B, O'Doherty J, Kaube H, Dolan RJ, Frith CD 2004b Empathy for pain involves the affective but not sensory components of pain. Science 303:1157–1162
Singer T, Seymour B, O'Doherty J, Stephan KE, Dolan RJ, Frith CD 2006 Empathic neural responses are modulated by the perceived fairness of others. Nature 439:466–469

Wicker B, Keysers C, Plailly J, Royet JP, Gallese V, Rizzolatti G 2003 Both of us disgusted in my insula: The common neural basis of seeing and feeling disgust. Neuron 40: 655–664

DISCUSSION

Frank: You mentioned the lack of prior work showing willingness to reward people who had behaved fairly. There is a paper by Kahneman and Thaler in which a group of people played a dictator game with two choices—five for the other person, five for yourself, or 10 for yourself and zero for the other person (Kahneman et al 1986). They recorded who did what in that game and gave a second group a chance to share $12 with the people who had been unfair in the first game, or $10 with the people who had been fair. Most people chose to take the lower reward that came with sharing money with the fairer people.

Singer: That's interesting.

Silk: I have a question about the last study you mentioned. I was wondering about the distribution of genders of the participants.

Singer: The gender in the first empathy study was randomly chosen. We used only women in the first study just because we wanted to fix a gender to control for possible gender effects. In the second study on modulation of empathy we then explicitly chose to test women and men to test for gender differences. In the last study on empathy for fairness we again tested only one gender, this time only men, because again we had to fix the gender to start with. However, we did a behavioural pilot study on women and men with the aim to determine whether men would punish more when the type of punishment is monetary points instead of pain. In this pilot study we didn't find any evidence for gender differences. Thus, I assume we will get similar results when testing women later.

Silk: Is there overall a difference in activation of these empathy-related responses between males and females?

Singer: I don't have brain data yet for the last study on empathic responses in third party games.

Silk: What about in the previous experiments you did, in the couples?

Singer: Again, with the couple I can't say, because I scanned only women. The only functional magnetic resonance imaging (fMRI) study I have done on gender differences in empathy is the one on modulation of empathy. In this one, we did not observe clear gender differences when men and women perceived a fair and likeable person in pain. However, we observed gender differences when a person who previously played unfairly received painful shocks. Then, men but not women showed an absence of empathic responses and an increase in activity in reward-related areas. The latter activity was correlated with their expressed desire for revenge as assessed after the study.

Hauser: In both papers we have heard so far I have been confused by the use of the term 'intention'. It seems different to the way the term is used in cognitive science. I have always been puzzled by this computer control. I understand that you get differences in activation when you are playing against the computer. If you tell someone they are playing against a human who plays completely randomly, versus a computer that plays strategically, do you still see differences in activation?

Singer: This hasn't been looked at, to my knowledge. In my study, however, in both cases the subjects think that they are playing against human playing partner, only that in one case these partners are told by a computer what to do and in the other case they are freely deciding what to do. The offers they get are identical in both conditions the only difference is the subjects' personal attribution of intentionality to the other players. But I see your point. You are saying that the relevant question is what sort of strategy are the subjects attributing to computers or to humans?

Hauser: When these systems are engaged, what is the nature of the object they are engaged with? There has been a blurring of the distinction between having the intention and having a goal. These are different things, but in this discussion they are being used interchangeably.

C Frith: We did an experiment on stone, paper, scissors where the subjects thought they were playing against a person or a computer. In this case we explicitly stated that the computer is using a very simple sequence that conceivably they might discover.

Hauser: What if you said that the person was doing the same thing? This is the key question.

Brosnan: In the study you mentioned you found a difference in whether the person you were scanning was male or female. Did it matter what gender the person they were playing with was? Did males react differently to males than females and so forth?

Singer: That's a good question. With our data set, however, we could not answer this question because we only had eight observations per cell and that is not enough to detect reliable differences. We tested for these gender differences but I would not draw any conclusion yet. Thus, for example activity in nucleus accumbens in men playing with women or men playing with men do not differ but the standard errors are also very big due to small sample size. We'd need a bigger study to look at this. There is a tendency for reliable gender differences in the attractiveness ratings. Women tend to find both female and male fair players very attractive and female and male unfair players very unattractive. Men show the same pattern for fair players, but tend to go less to the unattractive range when rating the attractiveness of unfair women players. That is, they still find bitches attractive albeit less than the cooperative ones!

Moll: Where does knowledge of the person, which actually drives decisions in these studies, fit in? You are mapping the outcome—the pay-off. In the first study the pain is applied to a person, and the subject in the scanner has a concept of this person. These fMRI designs clearly highlight differences in the limbic–paralimbic regions related to affective components, but don't tell us where the knowledge about the person is stored. This is, because when you compare say, the 'bad' person with the 'good one' directly, all fMRI responses to the representation of 'person' that you might know more or less well are wiped out. It would be interesting to see how empathic responses interact with the more large scale network, which probably includes the anterior temporal lobes and medial and lateral sectors of the orbitofrontal cortex, which are typically recruited by moral judgments (Moll et al 2005, de Quervain et al 2004). As a control, you could use the mere presence of this person. You could show a picture the face of the person.

Singer: This is essentially what I did in the first study published in *Neuron* on brain correlates underlying the moral status of faces in which I showed subjects faces of people who had previously played fair and unfairly (Singer et al 2004).

Moll: Exactly. And in that study, you found additional responses in the orbitofrontal cortex when comparing cooperators or non-cooperators to the faces of 'neutral' subjects, is that correct? I wonder if you compared the faces of cooperators, non-cooperators and neutral ones to a lower baseline, you would show the more ample prefronto–temporal network. It would be interesting then to explore how the representation of unique 'classes' of persons, potentially encoded in temporal cortex structures associated with semantic memory, would interact with the prefrontal cortex and paralimbic cortex, thereby integrating person knowledge with value representations. In fact, this is a prediction of our recent model of moral cognition (Moll et al 2005), in which a reputation of a person would involve the concept of 'fair' or 'unfair', linked to the representation of that person.

Singer: In this study I did not test for effects of situational context given the social situation of game play was used beforehand to build up a reputation of a fair and an unfair player. We then only tested implicit brain responses when subjects perceived the faces of these people who previously behaved fairly or unfairly in a social context. You could say that we measured brain networks subserving value judgement based on stored information about this person.

Moll: When you showed those effects, which was the baseline condition?

Singer: In this study we contrasted either faces of cooperative and defective subjects with neutral faces (they had engaged in games before which had no fair or unfair decision attached to them) or compared faces of players who had been intentionally involved in game play or told by a computer what to offer. The latter contrasts are even more conservative because in both cases faces had been previously associated with the same amount of winning or loosing money, the only difference between these conditions was whether subject attributed intentionality or not to their decisions. Interestingly, we saw in this study that a brain network associated with social cognition lighted up for intentional cooperators compared to non-intentional cooperators. Most strikingly the posterior superior temporal sulcus (STS) reacted only to the intentional but not to the non-intentional conditions. Thus, when perceiving an intentional fair or unfair agent enhanced activity in posterior STS could be observed. This was, however, not the case when perceiving neutral agents or agents whom you could not attribute any intentionality.

Montague: I'd like to make one comment, which is that the brain is a really complicated computational system. It would be shocking if every software domain in cognitive science had a one-to-one mapping on neural responses. There will be software levels where one level is hidden from the next, at least. For example, when you use your word processor it is the rules of what documents are and the rules of the package such as Microsoft Word, but underneath that is a program and operating system. There are layered connections. Attributing intentions to others is a software space that may not have a fixed place in the brain that is always being accessed. It may be floating around.

Moll: I'm just wondering why the anterior temporal lobe didn't show up during these interactions. This is probably an important region for the storage of semantic information about persons and functional concepts.

Montague: I don't know. I don't have an easy answer.

C Frith: I think it likely that the anterior temporal lobe was activated in both conditions. So it was 'subtracted out' in the comparison.

Singer: In this task, subjects didn't have to make any explicit judgement about the attribute of someone.

Moll: Semantic knowledge is typically activated automatically, in many instances even subconsciously. If you look at someone you know, the mere presence of this person, even if you are not explicitly thinking of her, then a very rich semantic and associative knowledge is implicitly activated (Caramazza & Mahon 2003, McClelland & Rogers 2003).

Montague: What does 'mere presence' mean?

Moll: When you see someone you know, you don't have to think explicitly about the features of that person. This is an important characteristic of semantic knowledge that can readily be used to make attributions about people.

Montague: To me this is not mere presence. The fact that you know them means that they are not merely present.

Moll: By 'mere presence', I just wanted to convey the idea that you don't need to make explicit judgments in order to engage social knowledge.

Montague: I don't know you, so if I saw a picture of you I'd have a very different response to the one I'd have if I saw my mother, which would induce a fear reaction in me!

Gallese: Coming back to empathy for pain, I have a question about the laterality of the activation of the insula. Do you systematically have a bilateral activation or does it tend to be more to the left or right?

Singer: I always see a bilateral activation of anterior insula in my studies. An interesting observation, however, is that the correlations with empathy questionnaires and AI—which I also replicated in the modulation of empathy study—tend to be always much more pronounced in the left AI. This is an interesting finding given the suggested importance of right AI for the representation of conscious feeling states.

Montague: These activations you get in the middle cingulate, bleeding up to the supplementary motor area, have been seen in pain studies, and are also seen when people do mental arithmetic.

Singer: The anterior cingulate cortex (ACC) is a very difficult brain area because first it is huge, second it is activated in a variety of different tasks and third even within pain processing different parts of the ACC are found to process different aspects of pain processing. Thus, intensity of pain seems to be processed more caudal whereas the emotional response to pain more rostral. Similarly, anterior insula (AI) is also involved in quite a variety of emotion-related tasks. Both, ACC and AI are probably subserving computational mechanisms which are very basic and domain general. They are also involved in the processing of pain, but that doesn't exclude that these regions also do something else.

Montague: The pain activation and mental arithmetic activation look almost exactly the same in our hands.

Hauser: Do you also get inferior parietal activation? This is a key area in studies of numerical quantification so we would expect to see activation.

Montague: It is the middle cingulate up into the supplementary motor area.

Singer: With regard to the observed activation in medial cingulate up into the supplementary motor areas it is noteworthy to state that this activation is in fact two different activations. In the first empathy study involving the couples the activation was so huge that the whole area was activated. If however, you have a look in the other empathy for pain studies which have now appeared this activation seems to be composed of two different peaks: a peak in premotor area and one in the ACC proper. This suggests that the premotor areas play a different role in pain processing than the ACC. Now another question. Is the mental arithmetic these people have done stressful or effortful? It is known that the ACC plays a key role in arousal and that the ACC probably has a more general role in integrating information about the autonomic nervous system to allow for effective motor behaviour, something like an alarm system of the brain. It might just be that the mental arithmetic is stressful and difficult and thus elicit arousal responses which in turn are computed by ACC.

Montague: We get them to subtract a number from 20, which is pretty simple.

Blair: I don't think that is a good argument with regards to the arousal data. You are basically saying that you have two indexes of conflict monitoring, one of which is ACC activity and the other which is the autonomic response. When you covary out the autonomic response you lose your ACC activation. But this doesn't necessarily mean that the ACC is generating autonomic signals. This result would be predicted if the ACC was only involved with conflict monitoring.

Singer: I agree. That is the common interpretation of the role of the ACC. And again, the ACC might act as a limbic motor cortex, as Bud Craig use to call it, and at the same time also do some very domain general processing such as coding for the intensity of painful stimulation. It's not all or none.

Blair: That seems to be a more sensible position. I wasn't sure whether you were trying to suggest that your pain empathy network and the fairness network are identical, and it is the same type of computational process, or that they just recruit the same neural regions to a greater or lesser extent? Or could it be that what we are picking up here is two systems that do a lot of things with respect to emotional processing? I can think of a few studies where both have come up simultaneously that have nothing to do with either empathy or fairness processing.

Singer: This is the big question. What is the general role of ACC and AI. Of course, there are no specific empathy or fairness areas. My view on this at the moment is that we have a brain response to the violation of fairness, which tags a system that is probably computing values in a more general sense. Bud Craig, Hugo Critchley, Antonio Damasio and others have recently suggested that the AI might be a 'interoceptive cortex' which subserves representations about bodily and feeling states. Thus, it is known to process pain, disgust and taste. It is involved in a lot of tasks which require subjective evaluation of feeling states, such as that feels good, that feels bad. According to such an interpretation the anterior cortex may play a crucial role in representing bodily states such as how aversive a certain pain felt for you but also for others. In the same vein it may also play a crucial role in processing aversive states elicited by the violation of implicit rules of fairness. Thus, if you feel treated unfairly you can easily feel a visceral body response of social disgust.

Blair: I don't think you need to limit it to body state. The insula will respond in decision making paradigms where the participant only receives greater or lesser amounts of points. It doesn't have to be body state reward or punishment. It could be that your position is that these two areas are both important emotional processing areas and emotional processing generally is involved in empathy and fairness calculations. The specific computations in both, however, could be completely different. In fact, there is a good chance they are different given the types of paradigms that are triggering a visual sight (in empathy) compared with the calculations (in fairness).

Singer: The input is clearly different, but if it is a value judgment in the sense of feels good/bad the output might be the same for both. It is coding a meaningful value about other people. I would love to make a single-cell recording in the human insula, but I have no idea where I would find these patients.

Van Lange: If you conceptualize some of your findings in terms of social pain, and compare them with physical pain, there are some differences in terms of how it affects the brain. One thing about social pain is that over time it may diminish, or there may be something like forgiveness. Do you have any plan to look at this over time? Over time the aversion to some pictures might diminish.

Singer: That is a good question. I have not looked into that at the moment. It is known however from research on amygdala functions that amygdala responses to the sight of perceiving aversive pictures or facial expressions of fear adapt over time.

Van Lange: It would be very dysfunctional if we were unable to forget or forgive over time. There are functional aspects to retaliation, as well. But forgiveness is also interesting because it could be functional too.

Singer: The only data I have on memory effects in the domain of social interactions and cheating are the behavioural data of the study published in *Neuron* on the acquired moral status of faces (Singer et al 2004). There I could show that after the experiment—that is, only two hours after having played with these people—memory is still better for cooperative or defecting people than for neutral ones. But of course this is short-term memory. You don't know how these effects would change over time and when confronted repeatedly with these people.

Dupoux: I have a comment about the finding that the pain system is also reacting to social pain. In your study you get the stronger response for the cooperator than the defector. In that sense, it is not only doing a different computational thing, but also the valence is very different.

Singer: That is a good point. Does the insula also compute different values? In the next study we will test for both dimensions—positive and negative. That is, we will include punishment and reward as well as fair and unfair offers. We want to see if we get different activation patterns for positive and negative values in the insula and ACC which would help to resolve this question.

Dupoux: Would you get empathy for pleasure also in these regions?

Singer: We don't know yet, but we are looking into this. At the moment, it seems that AI is processing both positive and negative feeling states. Thus, I observe AI activations for cooperation and for pain and others have found insula to be involved in positive and negative emotional states. In the literature, however, it is usually cited in association with negative states such as disgust and pain, but I don't think this is true. I think the insula has a much more general role in computing values. The interesting questions is now, whether different areas of the insula are computing different values or whether the story is much more complicated than that.

De Vignemont: In all your studies, the subjects were aware that the person in pain was not themselves, but someone else. Did you find any activation that could correspond to a distinction between self and other?

Singer: The group around Jean Decety, especially Perrine Ruby, has shown parietal activation in conditions that were meant to distinguish between attribution of mental states to self and other. In my studies I have an activation which I never know whether to call S2 or not. In some maps it is S2 and in some it isn't. It is bilateral activation in both studies on the edge of S2 and parietal areas. It is clearly not the contralateral S2 of the pain matrix. Thus, this activation might be associated with the ability to distinguish between self and other. But this would be purely speculative at this point.

Moll: Do you think that even when you make self/other distinctions, you might draw knowledge from the same representations of social knowledge? This would be more compatible with the mirror neuron story, and is economically interesting because you wouldn't need to have multiple representations for the same type of knowledge.

Singer: According to this view you would have the same networks activated but the magnitude of activation for example would serve as a tag for whether you or someone else is experiencing a state.

Moll: Yes. However, this distinction between self and other might only be possible at a conscious level, not by way of a single brain region, but from complex binding of very complex networks. In fact, no single focal lesions have been able to erase the sense of self.

C Frith: People with schizophrenia can sometimes get a bit confused about which is self and which is other.

Singer: The question about how the brain distinguishes between representation for self and others is indeed intriguing. What actually do you represent in ACC and anterior insula, the network activated when empathizing with the pain of others? Is it the representation of your own pain which you use to understand what it feels for others to be in pain? That would mean that empathy is biased on your own experience of pain and you just run this egocentric model to understand the outside world. Imagine, for example, what would happen if I see a masochist receiving pain and I knew that he indeed feels this stimulation as rewarding. Would then the reward network rather than my pain network light up in my brain? Probably not. There is probably an egocentricity bias in empathy in that you attribute states to the others who match your own previously acquired experiences. If you, for example, get analgesic medication so that you don't feel your pain anymore, probably you would then also show less of an activation in your pain network when perceiving another experiencing a similar painful stimulation. The question here is whether you are able to distinguish between your own values and those of others, that is represent the pain of others irrespective of what you are feeling?

Spinrad: I have a question that relates to both the mirror neuron work and yours. You have some evidence that the relational history with whomever it is that you are being empathic with plays a role. This is important in our work with toddlers, where we find that there are differences depending on who is the victim, and whether this is someone you have a relationship history with or someone who is a stranger (Spinrad & Stifter 2006). Are there differences that predict whether your empathy to another will differ on the basis of relationship history? There is some evidence in work with toddlers that socialization may play a stronger role in empathy towards someone with whom you have a relationship history (i.e. the mother; Robinson et al 2001). In contrast, genetic factors may play a stronger role in predicting empathy toward a stranger (Robinson et al 2001). For example, in a recent twin study, findings showed stronger evidence of genetic effects in empathy towards strangers, whereas there seems to be more environmental effects when predicting empathy toward the mother (Robinson et al 2001).

C Frith: I would like to go back to the general question of mirror neurons, and your assertion that their function may even be more specific than that. If you believe that these mirror systems are automatic and mandatory, this means that whenever we are walking around we are unconsciously responding to everything that we see people doing around us. These seems to me to be a little bit unlikely. There is an experiment by Janet Bavelas (Bavelas et al 1986) in which the subject is sitting in a waiting room waiting to do the experiment. Then two people bring in a heavy television set and one drops it on his finger. This is all videoed. If the TV handlers looking the other way, the subject looks with great curiosity and might raise her eyebrows. But if the person who drops the TV on his finger happens to be looking at the subject, then the subject shows a huge empathic change of expression. Perhaps these mirror systems are being switched on and off all the time depending on whether or not we are interacting with people.

Gallese: I would like to qualify better what I mean by 'mandatory' mechanism. Let's focus on mirror activation related to the observation of action. If the monkey doesn't pay attention to what is going on in front of it there is no response. The social stimulus has to be in the focus of attention. If this happens, the activation is automatic.

C Frith: I would go further and suggest that it is not only paying attention that matters, but also feeling that you are in some sort of social interaction with the other person.

Gallese: I would like to add something about the relationship between the personal history of an individual and the way this mirror mechanism is activated, not in the domain of emotion but in the domain of action. There is growing evidence that the way in which the system activates when you observe someone else acting is strongly influenced by your own motor experience. I'm thinking about the nice experiment done by Patrick Haggard and colleagues on dance observation in classic ballet and capoeira dancers (Calvo-Merino et al 2005). This study shows that if you are skilled in one kind of dance, you recognize it as more familiar. This recognition is somehow underpinned by a higher degree of activation of your own motor system. I suspect the same may apply to the domain of emotion.

Blakemore: I have a related question about the distinction between the mirror neuron system and the pain empathy system. There is no evidence that you can turn off your mirror neuron system for action, but you have shown that at least men can turn off their empathy for pain system. Is the distinction one of some kind of bottom–up versus top–down control? The question has been raised as to whether or not one is socially interacting when a person determines whether one shows mirror responses. But the fact that there are lots of premotor and other motor areas activated just by a subject seeing videos of hands grasping suggests that social interaction isn't needed for a mirror neuron response to action.

Singer: For pain it is the same. The mere perception of videos showing needles pricking a hand cause pain networks to be activated.

Blakemore: The question is, could you ever turn off the premotor cortex activation for the observation of action?

Singer: That's a good question.

Silk: I am wondering whether it could be interesting to look at these empathy responses to pain, not only responses to perception to what is fair or unfair, but also the perception of the punishing individual. If someone punishes someone for doing something that is wrong, they are doing something right in a moral world but something that causes pain. In a sense, it reverses the moral valence of the painful act. It is interesting from a theoretical view because punishment is rare in other species, but we humans have a real affinity for it. Where does this come from and how is it working?

C Frith: I thought Tania's experiment addressed this to an extent. It becomes right to punish an evil, unfair person.

Silk: But in punishing the person you are doing something in line with your own emotions about what that person has done.

Blair: I have a comment about the importance of the person paying attention for the mirror system to operate. It would be sad to forget the communicatory function of facial expressions and all the lovely Fridlund data (Fridlund 1991). These show that if you have a subject and then introduce someone into the room to interact with them, the subject shows lots more communication as a facial affect. This has nothing to do with mirror neurons.

C Frith: Does this mean that facial expressiveness is actively switched off when one is not communicating?

Blair: It seems to be pretty automatic. However, the use of facial expressions can also be goal directed.

Gallese: If we look at the literature on embodiment in social psychology, there is plenty of evidence showing that even if the information you are dealing with is totally remote from the real target of the experiment—say you are reading stuff about the elderly people and you are supposed to rate the orthographic correctness of the style, then it takes you longer to get out of the building compared with people who are primed with material related to a more athletic subject. This shows that the activation of an embodied mechanism is something that we are most of the time totally unaware of. Therefore we have no control of it.

Hauser: I have been thinking about an experiment that might help us with mirror neurons. What happens to the mirror neurons when you are watching yourself in the mirror? The reason for asking is that you are watching your own motor system. Can you get to a point where you know it is happening? Can you turn the system off and what happens to the system? The system is getting double input. There is no sense that early in development the mirror system is active, but infants do imitation very early on, yet they don't have mirror self recognition. To what extent would information on mirrors tell you something about the mandatoriness of the mechanism and about the top–down aspects?

Gallese: That is a good point. No one knows.

References

Bavelas JB, Black A, Lemery CR, Mullett J 1986 I show how you feel—motor mimicry as a communicative act. J Personal Social Psychol 50:322–329

Calvo-Merino B, Glaser DE, Grezes J, Passingham RE, Haggard P 2005 Action observation and acquired motor skills: an fMRI study with expert dancers. Cereb Cortex 8:1243–1249

Caramazza A, Mahon BZ 2003 The organization of conceptual knowledge: the evidence from category-specific semantic deficits. Trends Cogn Sci 7:354–3615

Fridlund AJ 1991 Sociality of solitary smiling: Potentiation by an implicit audience. J Personal Social Psychol 60:229–246

de Quervain DJ, Fischbacher U, Treyer V et al 2004 The neural basis of altruistic punishment. Science 305:1246–1247

Kahneman D, Knetsch J, Thaler R 1986 Fairness and the assumptions of economics. J Business 59:S285–300

McClelland JL, Rogers TT 2003 The parallel distributed processing approach to semantic cognition. Nat Rev Neurosci 4:310–322

Moll J, Zahn R, de Oliveira-Souza R, Krueger F, Grafman J 2005 Opinion: the neural basis of human moral cognition. Nat Rev Neurosci 6:799–809

Robinson JL, Zahn-Waxler C, Emde RN 2001 Relationship context as a moderator of sources of individual difference in empathic development. In: Emde RN, Hewitt JK (eds) Infancy to early childhood: genetic and environmental influences on developmental change). Oxford University Press, Oxford, p 257–268

Singer T, Kiebel SJ, Winston JS, Dolan RJ, Frith CD 2004 Brain responses to the acquired moral status of faces. Neuron 41:653–662

Spinrad TL, Stifter CA 2006 Empathy-related responding to distress in toddlers: predictions from negative emotionality and maternal behaviour in infancy. Infancy, in press

What's fair? The unconscious calculus of our moral faculty

Marc Hauser

Departments of Psychology, Organismic & Evolutionary Biology, and Biological Anthropology, Harvard University, Cambridge, MA 02138, USA

Abstract. This essay argues that much of the research in moral psychology has focused on moral performance, on what people do. The study of moral competence, in contrast, has largely been ignored. I use the analogy to linguistics as a model for exploring our moral competence, and suggest that we are endowed with a moral faculty that operates over the causes and consequences of actions. This moral faculty is endowed with principles and parameters that are universal. Acquiring a particular moral system entails setting the parameters. On this model, emotions such as empathy are consequences (as opposed to causes) of unconscious but principled moral evaluations.

2006 Empathy and Fairness. Wiley, Chichester (Novartis Foundation Symposium 278) p 41–55

The famine crisis in Bangladesh covered the airwaves and papers in the 1960s and early 1970s. To keep the Bengali refugees alive for one year would have cost the world approximately 750 million dollars. Britain was one of the major contributors, giving about 25 million dollars in one year. This may seem like a healthy contribution for one nation, but in that same year, Britain contributed close to 500 million dollars to help the French build the Concorde jet. As Peter Singer (1972) remarked 'the British government values a supersonic transport more than thirty times as highly as it values the lives of nine million refugees.'

The situation today is hardly better. The World Bank estimated that out of approximately 6 billion people on earth in the year 2000, almost half fell below the poverty line. Poverty translates not only to hunger, but illnesses and insufficient medical aid. In 2005, the United Nation's World Food Programme projected that it would cost just over 3 billion dollars to feed 73 million hungry people, leaving an additional 800 million people in a state of starvation. Providing relief for the remaining numbers, and ending world hunger for 2005, would run the globe an additional 35 billion dollars, bringing the tab up to about 40 billion dollars. The USA spends about 40 billion dollars each year on gambling, a superfluous activity that no one needs. If everyone stayed away from the slot machines and poker tables for just one year, voila, hunger relief for all.

We spend equally vast amounts of money on other superfluous activities including dieting programmes, entertainment, unnecessarily large vehicles and toys for our children. Wouldn't the fair thing be to convert our frivolity into lives saved?

When statistics such as these are trotted out without labelling the countries—for example, in response to country A's need for $500 million in relief funds, country B gave $10 million but also spent $800 million on the production of a single blockbuster movie—it is hard to imagine anyone having the intuition that such policies of resource distribution are permissible or fair. In fact, it seems down and out wrong—morally wrong that is. Why then has the situation remained unchanged? Why are we so incapable of doing the morally right thing? Why do our intuitions fire one way and our actions another? The argument that I develop here is that when we deliver moral judgments, we do so on the basis of unconscious, intuitive biases—operative principles that are often disconnected with the complicated processes that ultimately lead to explicit actions and often, post-hoc justifications.

In a discussion of famine relief, Singer (1972) provides a simple principle to guide the psychology of obligatory aid [p 229]: *If it is in our power to prevent something bad from happening, without thereby sacrificing anything of comparable moral importance, we ought, morally, to do it.* What is crucial about the *Singer principle* is that it links the psychology of moral obligation up with the cold calculus of cost–benefit analysis and the systems of motivation. And it creates this link without making reference to a particular group of people and their relationship to the morally responsible agent; it is an impartial moral principle. Nothing in the Singer principle depends upon whether the individual or individuals in need are neighbours or foreigners, near or far. Further, nothing hangs on whether there are one or more potential contributing agents to the cause. Everything hangs, however, on the phrase 'without sacrificing anything of comparable moral importance.' This is a sticky phrase, one that has constantly confronted utilitarians such as Singer. The stickiness is due to one word—*comparable*—and its frame of reference—*comparable* to what standard and whose standards? When we think about fairness, we evaluate the distribution of resources—either concrete property or more abstract rights—based on some standard and based on some sense of value, of doing what is best for some set of relevant others.

To highlight the challenge of making this principle do some real work, and to see how it pushes our sense of what is fair, consider the following three cases.

Case 1: Are we morally obligated to give money to an aid organization to purchase rehydration salts for children in sub-Saharan Africa instead of buying a candy bar? Saving one or more children from death due to dehydration is unquestionably worth the personal sacrifice of junk sugar. Our moral calculus should compel our motivational systems to act and do the morally right and virtuous thing: give to the aid organization. Here we push against the problem of temporal discounting (Ainslie 2000, Elster 2000), and the challenge of bypassing the short-term but small benefit for the delayed but large benefit for both self and other.

Case 2: What about our moral obligation to fund the relief program in Case 1 instead of sending our children to college? Our children don't *need* an education for survival. Four years of college tuition at the Ivy League Schools in the year 2005 exceeded $200000 for one student, a sum that would do wonders for relief programmes. But knowledge is a great thing to own, and colleges make this possible. Everyone, universally, agrees that education is important. But few, if any, think that an education is more important than surviving. If I had to put money into my daughter's college tuition or relieve her of a medical problem, there would be no contest: medical relief.

Case 3: consider the classic trolley problems, initially raised by Phillipa Foot (1967), in which our moral psychology is asked to adjudicate on the extent to which it is permissible to harm another if we can potentially save many more. In one scenario, a bystander can prevent five people from being run over by an out of control trolley by flipping a switch; flipping the switch turns the trolley onto a side track where it kills one person. In a second scenario, a bystander can push a heavy man in front of the trolley; the trolley runs over and kills the heavy man, but stops before it hits the five. Most people think it is permissible to flip the switch, but forbidden to push the man. In seeing the switch case as permissible, we see one person's life as less important than five. Using the Singer principle, it is in the agent's power to prevent something bad from happening (killing 5), without thereby sacrificing anything of comparable moral importance (one life is not as important as five lives); therefore, the agent ought, morally, to flip the switch. In the pushing case, we flip the argument around, essentially saying that one person's life is of equal (or greater) moral importance compared to five people's lives, and thus, we should not push the man. Filling in the principle, it is in the agent's power to prevent something bad from happening (killing 5), but killing 1 entails sacrificing something of comparable moral importance and thus, the agent ought not, morally, to push the man. As stated, the Singer principle can't arbitrate between these cases. How do we decide what counts as comparable in 'moral importance?' Are we missing the essential parameters that modulate the outcome of our decision? Should we allow for a liberal plurality of views under some circumstances? No easy answers here.

The discussion of world hunger raises the competence–performance distinction, a fundamental contrast between our intuitive moral judgments and our actual moral actions. We may all judge, spontaneously, with no reflection, that it is permissible to provide aid to children lacking dehydration salts, but when it comes to writing our cheques, we balk, for one or more reasons. The Singer principle is an idealization of what we ought to do. It is a beautifully simple and clear prescriptive principle. It is of course possible that at some level of abstraction it is also a descriptive principle that is part of our moral psychology. Everyone, it seems, has the intuition that cost-free rescue is morally obligatory: we must save a drowning baby from a bathtub even if we get wet, and we must give our candy bar to a starving child even if we were looking forward to a yummy snack. These situations are easy, and the idealized principle works beautifully. But the world is ugly. From the triggering of something like the Singer principle to the implementation of an action, there are many mind internal and external processes that intervene and contribute to our behaviour including the motivational and cost-benefit systems, as well as the empathic response that is yanked from many of us at the sight of starving children, a drowning baby, or an individual in harm's way of a runaway trolley.

These are hard problems. They have been debated for decades among philosophers, politicians, lawyers, lobbyists and presumably countless families eating dinner in the developed world. They raise fundamental challenges for each of us as we contemplate the ingredients that enter into a moral life. What I wish to do in the remaining sections of this essay is showcase how we might approach the problem of moral evaluation from an empirical perspective, driven by a theoretical framework that has been frequently entertained, but never seriously explored. It is a framework that takes as a starting point the competence–performance distinction raised above, noting that there are fundamental differences between the unconscious operative principles that drive our intuitive judgments and the expressed judgments that we articulate in an attempt to justify our actions. It is a framework that builds on John Rawls' (1971) early articulation of justice as fairness, and especially, his use of an analogy to language to formulate the proper level of description of our moral faculty.

I first provide a sketch of this view of our moral faculty—of a Rawlsian creature equipped with a suite of universal moral principles that operate over the causes and consequences of action. I then contrast the Rawlsian creature with two others, the logical, rational, and consciously principled Kantian and the emotional, intuitive Humean. The goal is to show that an empirical science of our moral psychology must consider these distinct processes, as well as the manner in which they potentially interact in guiding our moral judgments and actions.

Model 1:

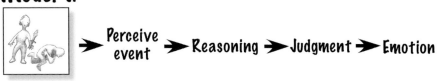

Perceive event → Reasoning → Judgment → Emotion

FIG. 1.   The Kantian creature and the deliberate reasoning model

Kantian, Humean and Rawlsian creatures

Rawls (1971) was interested in the idea that the principles underlying our intuitions about morality may well be unconscious and inaccessible[1]. This perspective was intended to parallel Chomsky's thinking in linguistics. Unfortunately, those writing about morality in neighbouring disciplines, especially within the sciences, held a different perspective. The then dominant position in developmental psychology, championed by Piaget (1932/1965) and Kohlberg (1981), was that the child's moral behaviour is best understood in terms of her capacity to articulate particular moral principles. On this view, children gradually develop into mini-Kantians (1785/1959, 2001), justifying their moral decisions by appealing to particular ethical principles that have universal acceptance. A morally mature child not only distinguishes between fair and unfair transactions, but appeals to principles of distributive justice to account for his/her decisions.

   Figure 1 captures the essence of the Piaget and Kohlberg perspective on moral judgment, and what I will characterize as the moral psychology of a Kantian creature (Hauser 2006): the perception of an event is followed by reasoning, which

---

[1] Rawls' views on the linguistic analogy are presented in section 9 of *A Theory of Justice*, but the precursor to this discussion originates in his thesis and the several papers that followed. For example, in his thesis he states [p 72–73] 'The meaning of explication may be stated another way: ordinarily the use of elaborate concepts is intuitive and spontaneous, and therefore like "cause", "event", "good", are applied intuitively or by habit, and not by consciously applied rules ... Sometimes, instead of using the term "explication" one can use the phrase "rational reconstruction" and one can say that a concept is rationally reconstructed whenever the correct rules are stated which enable one to understand and explain all the actual occasions of its use.' Further on, he states [p 107] that moral principles are 'analogous to functions. Functions, as rules applied to a number, yield another number. The principles, when applied to a situation yield a moral rule. The rules of common sense morality are examples of such secondary moral rules.' See Mikhail for a more comprehensive discussion of Rawls' linguistic analogy, together with several important extensions.

results in a judgment; emotion may emerge from the judgment, but is not causally related to it. Here, actions are evaluated by reflecting upon specific principles, and using this reflective process to rationally deduce a specific judgment. When we deliver a moral verdict it is because we have considered different possible reasons for and against a particular action, and based on this deliberation, alight upon a particular decision. Although Kant never denied the role of intuition in the process of moral deliberation, he, more than many other moral philosophers, emphasized the role of rational deliberation about what one ought to do.

The Piaget/Kohlberg tradition has provided rich and reliable data on the moral stages through which children pass, using their justifications as primary evidence for developmental change. In recent years, however, a number of cognitive and social psychologists have criticized this perspective (Macnamara 1990), especially its insistence that the essence of moral psychology is *justification* rather than *judgment*. It has been observed that even fully mature adults are sometimes unable to provide any sufficient justification for strongly felt moral intuitions, a phenomenon termed 'moral dumbfounding' (Haidt 2001). This has led to the introduction of a second model, characterized most recently by Haidt (2001) as well as several other social psychologists and anthropologists (Fig. 2). Here, following the perception of an action or event, there is an unconscious emotional response which immediately causes a moral judgment, reasoning is an afterthought, offering a post-hoc rationalization of an intuitively generated response. We see someone standing over a dead person and we classify this as murder, a claim that derives from a pairing between any given action and a classification of morally right or wrong; a parallel case is imagined for helping, with sympathy or empathy driving the show. Emotion triggers the judgment. I call this model 'Humean', after the philosopher who famously declared that reason is 'slave to the passions'.

A second recent challenge to the Piaget/Kohlberg tradition is a hybrid between the Humean and Kantian creatures, a blend of unconscious emotions and some form of principled and deliberate reasoning (Fig. 3); this view has most recently been championed by Damasio based on neurologically impaired patients (Anderson et al 1999, Damasio 1994, Tranel et al 2000) and by Greene based on

Model 2:

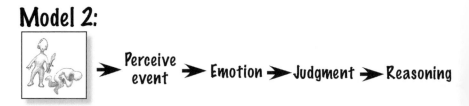

FIG. 2.   The Humean creature and the emotional model.

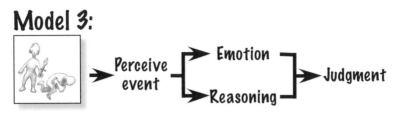

FIG. 3.   A mixture of the Kantian and Humean creatures, blending the reasoning and emotional models

neuroimaging work (Greene et al 2001, 2004). These two systems may converge or diverge in their assessment of the situation, run in parallel or in sequence, but both are precursors to the judgment; if they diverge, then some other mechanism must intrude, resolve the conflict and generate a judgment. On Damasio's view, every moral judgment includes both emotion and reasoning. On Greene's view, emotions come into play in situations of a more personal nature, and favour more deontological judgments, while reason comes into play in situations of a more impersonal nature, and favours more utilitarian judgments.

Independently of which account turns out to be correct, this breakdown reveals a missing ingredient in almost all current theories and studies of our moral psychology. It will not do merely to assign the role of moral judgment to reason, emotion or both. We must describe computations underlying the judgments that we produce. In contrast to the detailed work in linguistics focusing on the principles that organize phonology, semantics and syntax, we lack a comparably detailed analysis of how humans and other organisms perceive actions and events in terms of their causes and consequences for self and other. As I (Hauser et al 2006a) and others (Dwyer 1999, 2004, Jackendoff 2005, Mikhail 2006) have noted, actions represent the right kind of unit for moral appraisal: discrete and combinable to create a limitless range of meaningful variation.

To fill in this missing gap, we must characterize knowledge of moral codes in a manner directly comparable to the linguist's characterization of knowledge of language. This insight is at the heart of Rawls' linguistic analogy. Rawls (1971) writes, 'A conception of justice characterizes our moral sensibility when the everyday judgments we make are in accordance with its principles.' He went on to sketch the connection to language:

A useful comparison here is with the problem of describing the sense of grammaticalness that we have for the sentences of our native language. In this case, the aim is to characterize the ability to recognize well-formed sentences by formulating clearly expressed principles which make the same discriminations as the native speaker. This is a difficult undertaking which, although still unfinished, is known to require theoretical constructions that far outrun the ad hoc precepts of our explicit grammatical knowledge. A similar situation presumably holds in moral philosophy. There is no reason to assume that our sense of justice can be adequately characterized by familiar common sense precepts, or derived from the more obvious learning principles. A correct account of moral capacities will certainly involve principles and theoretical constructions which go beyond the norms and standards cited in every day life (p 46–47).

With these ideas in place, we are ready to introduce the *Rawlsian creature*, equipped with the machinery to deliver moral verdicts based on principles that may be inaccessible (Fig. 4); in fact, if the analogy to language holds, the principles will be operative but not expressed, and only discoverable with the tools of science. There are two ways to view the Rawlsian creature in relationship to the other models. Minimally, each of the other models must recognize an appraisal system that computes the causes and consequences of actions. More strongly, the Rawlsian creature provides the sole basis for our judgments of morally forbidden, permissible or obligatory actions, with emotion and reasoning following in their wake. To be clear: the Rawlsian model does not deny the role of emotion or reasoning. Rather, it stipulates that any process giving rise to moral judgments must minimally do so on the basis of some system of analysis, and that this analysis constitutes the heart of the moral faculty. On the stronger view, the operative principles of the moral faculty do all the heavy lifting, generating a moral verdict that may or may not produce an emotion or a process of rational and principled deliberation. If this view is correct, then it makes a series of testable predictions. Neuroimaging studies with sufficiently good temporal and spatial resolution should reveal that the circuitry involved in emotional processing activates after we deliver a moral judgment. Similarly, patients with damage to this circuitry should show normal patterns of moral judgements, given that emotions are triggered in response to these judgments. Finally, if the appraisal system is associated with our moral competence, but our emotions play their most significant role in our moral actions, then we would expect to find patients that provide normal judgments but act inappropriately. Psychopaths are the most likely candidates. Tests using neuroimaging and patient populations are currently underway.

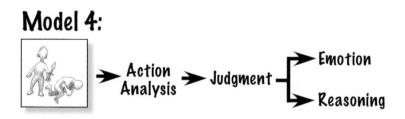

FIG. 4.   The Rawlsian creature and action analysis model.

My goal here has been to make a convincing case for considering each of these processes. The Rawlsian creature has been a neglected species in our attempt to understand the nature of our moral judgments. But putting this perspective on the table is critical, as important as Chomsky's parallel formulation of the problem in linguistics. If we don't distinguish between competence and performance, as well as operative and expressed principles, we will be arguing past each other. We will also miss out on a description of the potential knowledge that all mature individuals bring to bear on their moral judgments, and how this knowledge grows in each individual and evolved within our species, perhaps uniquely. Importantly, the issues raised by this perspective are highly testable, as recent work with normal subjects, cross-cultural populations, brain damaged patients and imaging technologies reveals (Hauser 2006, Hauser et al 2006a, b, Mikhail et al 1998, Mikhail 2000, 2006). Much of our recent work shows that when people, from different ages, cultures, religious backgrounds and educations, judge cases involving helping and harming others, they do so in a relatively uniform, and universally shared way. They also do so without access to the underlying principles. These results raise the possibility of a universal moral grammar, a signature of our species.

References

Ainslie G 2000 Break-down of will. Cambridge University Press, New York

Anderson SW, Bechara A, Damasio H, Tranel D, Damasio AR 1999 Impairment of social and moral behavior related to early damage in human prefrontal cortex. Nat Neurosci 2: 1032–1037

Damasio A 1994 Descartes' error. Norton, Boston, MA

Dwyer S 1999 Moral competence. In: Murasugi K & Stainton R (eds) Philosophy and linguistics. Westview Press, Boulder p 169–190

Dwyer S 2004 How good is the linguistic analogy. Retrieved February 25, from www.umbc. edu/philosophy/dwyer

Elster J 2000 Ulysses unbound. Cambridge University Press, New York

Foot P 1967 The problem of abortion and the doctrine of double effect. Oxford Review 5: 5–15

Greene JD, Nystrom LE, Engell AD, Darley JM, Cohen JD 2004 The neural bases of cognitive conflict and control in moral judgment. Neuron 44:389–400

Greene JD, Sommerville RB, Nystrom LE, Darley JM, Cohen JD 2001 An fMRI investigation of emotional engagement in moral judgment. Science 293:2105–2108

Haidt J 2001 The emotional dog and its rational tail: A social intuitionist approach to moral judgment. Psychol Rev 108:814–834

Hauser MD 2006 Moral minds: the unconscious voice of right and wrong. Harper Collins, New York

Hauser MD, Cushman F, Young L 2006a Reviving Rawls' linguistic analogy: operative principles and the causal structure of moral actions. In: W. Sinnott-Armstrong (ed), Moral psychology and biology. Oxford University Press, New York, in press

Hauser MD, Cushman F, Young L, Jin RK-X, Mikhail J 2006b A dissociation between moral judgment and justification. Mind and language, in press

Jackendoff R 2005 Language, culture, consciousness: Essays on mental structure. In: (ed) MIT Press, Cambridge

Kant I 1785/1959 Foundations of the metaphysics of morals. Macmillan, New York

Kant I 2001 Lectures on ethics. Cambridge University Press, New York

Kohlberg L 1981 Essays on moral development, Volume 1: The philosophy of moral development. Harper Row, New York

Macnamara J 1990 The development of moral reasoning and the foundations of geometry. J Theor Soc Behav 21:125–150

Mikhail J 2000 Rawls' linguistic analogy: A study of the 'generative grammar' model of moral theory described by John Rawls in 'A theory of justice'. Unpublished PhD, Cornell University, Ithaca

Mikhail J 2006 Rawls' linguistic analogy. Cambridge University Press, New York, in press

Mikhail J, Sorrentino C, Spelke ES 1998 Toward a universal moral grammar. Paper presented at the Proceedings of the Cognitive Science Society

Piaget J 1932/1965 The moral judgment of the child. Free Press, New York

Rawls J 1971 A theory of justice. Harvard University Press, Cambridge

Singer P 1972 Famine, affluence, and morality. Philos Public Aff 1/3:229–243

Tranel D, Bechara A, Damasio A 2000 Decision making and the somatic marker hypothesis. In: Gazzaniga M (ed) The new cognitive neurosciences. MIT Press, Cambridge p 1047–1061

DISCUSSION

C Frith: When you were talking about people with orbitofrontal damage, the argument seemed to be that these people don't have emotion. What do you really think is wrong?

Hauser: I would argue that there is an emotional deficit that links to decision-making. If you don't have that link, there will be problems with your decision-making process. If this is true, and you do need the emotional connections to make decisions about the moral sphere, then they should look abnormal. The point is, they don't in many cases. The job is to provide a more nuanced view about the nature of that deficit, which is how various aspects of emotion may connect up with certain kinds of decisions.

C Frith: I was thinking of the recent work on anticipated regret, which goes into much more detail about the precise relationship between the kind of emotion and its relevance to decision making (Camille et al 2004). It would be interesting to analyse some of those scenarios in terms of this.

Call: Have you looked for individual differences?

Hauser: This is a huge sample size where the proportions are often monumental. There are individual differences. In these particular cases, some people don't see a difference. Many people have given us their e-mail address, so we can go back to them and ask them more questions. For example, in some action–omission cases, people say that they just don't want to take the responsibility. Of course, by not omitting an action, they are taking responsibility. The point is, that action–omission bias is a monumental one in our psychology which comes up in all sorts of aspects of behaviour. In euthanasia, for example, for many people mercy killing is not OK but letting die is.

Call: Can you see some profiles of certain groups of individuals?

Hauser: Classically, people that take the 'no responsibility' view stick with it until you push them hard, for example by saying that their mother is on the track. You can see that they are holding onto these kinds of views. We haven't looked carefully into individual variation. I am looking for the majority response and using this as a way of getting at what might be the universal moral psychology.

De Vignemont: I am a little worried that the replies that you get depend on the question that you ask. If you ask *what is worst,* killing the fat guy or killing the hiker, then subjects might reply that it is worst when it is the hiker. Indeed, his death was meaningless because it did not help to save the other people, it was merely an after-effect, while the fat guy's death is meaningful because at least it was able to save the other person. Such question may appeal more to the emotional system. In contrast, when you ask *what is permissible,* you appeal more to rationality or reasoning, and may end up with a different answer.

Hauser: There is no point of disagreement here. It is like in linguistics: I can either probe pragmatics or syntax. You can engage different parts of the brain. It is certainly interesting to see whether we can prime the utilitarian perspective. How penetrable is this system, and how penetrable are these principles? Here's a way in which morality and language may be very different. Let's say that we uncover some unconscious and inaccessible principle and all of a sudden we begin writing about it in the popular press. Now people begin to think about their actions in terms of this principle. Will it affect their behaviour? The fact that Noam Chomsky has deeper insights into language than I do, doesn't make him a better speaker or writer. This may not be true for the moral faculty. It may be that the principles are impenetrable, but once they are raised into our awareness and discussed, they can affect behaviour. This is why the religious work is interesting because these are people who in their responses are frequently very religious, but this doesn't change their judgements or justifications. If you are a believer, or not, you generate similar moral judgments in these contexts.

Dupoux: You took the analogy of language. In the case of language you have universal principles and also variation across language. You showed data describing ideas of what could be universal parameters. What would the variation be? Will there be any?

Hauser: Yes. In the same way that some people might want to argue that things like the computation merge in language is universal, there may be core computations in morality that are also universal. The question is, what are the parametric variations? There is fascinating work by Phil Tetlock at the University of California, Berkeley, that reveals certain kinds of trade-offs between actions with different payoffs. In brief, there are some exchanges that people just don't allow because they are morally offensive and thus, taboo. For example, let's say that I come to you and say 'I know you have a daughter, and I want to give you $1 million for your daughter'. You reject my offer. Being persistent, I up the offer to $1 billion. The longer you delay your response to my offer, contemplating the possibility of an exchange, the more you feel a sense of moral corruption, even disgust. It may be that everyone universally has a taboo of exchanges, but the content of that exchange is what can vary cross-culturally. People could have a universal sense of fairness of exchange, and the parameter could be what is traded. This is where variation could come in. If the analogy to language is applicable, though, people are thinking about this in the wrong way. They are at the surface level of moral behaviour, and haven't looked at the architecture in the right way, peering under the surface to look at what is operative in terms of principles even if they are not expressed. My strong sense is that a principle like the doctrine of double effect is much too coarse grain and that we will need to look at more abstract psychological distinctions and how they interact to generate the causes and consequences that yield moral judgments.

Gergely: Following the linguistic analogy, in language universal grammar has a developmental aspect: it functions as a language acquisition device. Is there something similar in morality? Also, what is the reason for the cognitive opacity of morality?

Hauser: I was surprised when I started looking at the developmental literature on morality. I asked a lot of people about this. To my knowledge, no one has raised seriously the idea of a critical period for moral acquisition. Everyone's intuition is that we acquire morality like language. There is no evidence or anything like data that bears on the pattern of acquisition of morality. My prediction would be that because it has surface-level similarities to language, children need very little input. People haven't done your kind of work either, looking at action in terms of its teleological patterning, and how these kinds of cognitive operations might be necessary steps into the moral sphere, even though they are clearly not unique to morality. On the evolutionary side you can imagine a system where every social norm was perfectly accessible to conscious thought. I think this would create grave difficulties for social functioning. I think that a system that is operatively automatic would be favourable. If you are constantly accessing the principles driving your behaviour, it would be like me thinking about my nouns, verbs and adjectives: I would never have a conversation. The question is whether this is unconscious in the school grammar sense of unconscious or in the Chomsky and linguistic sense.

Frank: It helps you act more quickly but it may help to commit you to act in certain ways that wouldn't be credible otherwise. You suggest that the emotions are more important for their influence on your behaviour than your judgement. If I am considering whether you are to be trusted, then what most interests me is what you will do if I send you to engage in a task where you could cheat me and I wouldn't know. If I can know you to experience those emotions, this is an important signal to me about whether you are to be trusted.

Hauser: So you are saying that if you knew that I was a person who experienced emotion, this is important information.

Frank: And it is advantageous for you that I should be able to know this.

Hauser: Absolutely. I am not saying that all these things don't figure into our moral behaviour. I am taking a view that here is a corner of our moral psychology that has not been investigated. How this corner interfaces with the other parts of the brain will be a complicated story. It is too big to think about at the moment.

Frank: The judgement does seem to follow the emotion at least in part. In my case, I feel my judgement in the examples you gave is influenced by the emotion I feel.

Hauser: This is where the history of intuitive psychology sends up a warning flag. We often have no intuitions or the wrong ones, so we must be careful about letting our intuitions drive what we think is an appropriate characterization of the underlying psychology. Here is the alternative challenge. I can imagine a principle which simply involves near and far as a parameter and has nothing to do with emotion. Actions that are near are treated differently to actions that are far.

Frank: If your mother is far away you would experience an emotion.

Hauser: Yes, but the question I am asking is whether it is this experience that drives the judgment. When you see your mother, you can't have the emotion until some system first classifies the person as your mother, and then this launches a cascade of associations, some to your emotions and some to other bits of data. But one could run the calculation in another, completely unemotional way. I code the situation first as near/far. I then code the target in terms of degrees of genetic relatedness. From this calculation, I generate a judgment. There is zero emotion in my description. This goes through and I get an answer. Then emotions follow. Imagine a completely cold calculus being in place. What kinds of empirical data would you use to arbitrate between these?

Blair: I disagree. The first thing you said was that you claimed the trolley examples to be emotionally equivalent. But they aren't. The Joshua Greene data show that the neural correlates of the emotional response distinguish between apparently equal levels of damage to one person versus another. You could say that is secondary, but then your argument that there is no emotion no longer holds. This leads us to the frontal cases. You were suggesting that in the more extreme examples you didn't need emotion in a sort of compromise position. But I suggest that this is not the correct compromise. The position I would hold is that if you are in those extreme examples, there is a strong emotional push to help him, and therefore even an individual who has a weak emotional response would show equivalent responding. Having said all this, this is clearly not the case with those patients.

They are clearly different. Rather than being less likely to help, they are more likely to help. This is consistent with the idea that these people are dysregulated from their basic emotional architecture. If this is true, the individuals with psychopathy will look strikingly different from the orbitofrontal cortex (OFC) patients in that they will be less likely to help. All the data you have presented are highly compatible with an emotion primacy position. This is not to say that there aren't input conditions that generate the level of emotional response. There are many ways of regulating the intensity of the emotional response, but these are input conditions and the emotional response is the important thing.

Hauser: The problem with Josh Greene's studies (Greene et al 2001, 2004) is that the dilemmas were not that well controlled in terms of the text, and the reaction time analyses pooled over the various kinds of dilemmas. What makes our work different is that we carefully control the text, using a template to clone each variant, systematically only changing one parameter or factor. In some of the key contrasts, there are no differences that link to emotion, but rather, to whether the consequences of the agent's actions were intended or foreseen.

Blair: There is nothing as regards to the level of victims that is different. The difference is that in one case we have an intentional action with a goal of squishing a person; in the other case my goal is to get the train blocked. I'm not even attending, necessarily, to the victim. My prediction would be that if you did an RT study looking at accessing the consequences of the action, people would be quite slow in accessing the consequences of the victim in the block example but fast in the other one. Those conditions aren't equivalent with regard to the emotional response.

Hauser: In some senses I agree. I think we don't know what role emotions are playing in these judgements. Until we proposed the linguistic analogy, following up on John Rawls' intuition in the 1970s and John Mikhail's thesis (Mikhail 2000), there were no alternatives; there was just the idea that emotions drive the judgements or it is consciously reasoned. At the moment there are no data that would allow us to distinguish which theoretical perspective is correct.

Blair: There are. There are the moral conventional distinction data, which is a moral reasoning task.

Hauser: I'm not saying that emotions can't modulate some of our moral decisions.

Blair: That is exactly what you said in your model.

Hauser: As we have discussed, the way you set up the moral conventional distinction is different from how we run our dilemmas, and they potentially tap different elements of the psychology. Moreover, there is certainly a growing perspective that the moral-conventional distinction as originally articulated by Turiel is less clear-cut than expressed, with many interesting discussions now ongoing. So I will still hold to the position that we lack the requisite data for distinguishing between the various explanations for the sources of our moral judgments.

C Frith: I thought the most interesting point you made is whether they will actually behave like this. I look forward greatly to seeing how these moral dilemmas will be put into real life. I think one of the interesting things about the studies of economic games is that here we have people in semi-real life situations behaving in fair and unfair ways and responding appropriately, rather than people making off-line judgements about what would be fair behaviour. It would be interesting to see whether the moral dilemmas could be put into game situations like this.

References

Camille N, Coricelli G, Sallet J, Pradat-Diehl P, Duhamel JR, Sirigu A 2004 The involvement of the orbitofrontal cortex in the experience of regret. Science 304:1167–1170

Greene JD, Nystrom LE, Engell AD, Darley JM, Cohen JD 2004 The neural bases of cognitive conflict and control in moral judgment. Neuron 44:389–400

Greene JD, Sommerville RB, Nystrom LE, Darley JM, Cohen JD 2001 An fMRI investigation of emotional engagement in moral judgment. Science 293:2105–2108

Mikhail JM 2000 Rawls' linguistic analogy: A study of the 'generative grammar' model of moral theory described by John Rawls in 'A theory of justice'. In: Philosophy. Cornell University, Ithaca, p 375

Chimpanzees may recognize motives and goals, but may not reckon on them

Josep Call and Keith Jensen

Max Planck Institute for Evolutionary Anthropology, Leipzig, Germany

Abstract. Psychological states play a fundamental role in mediating human social interactions. We interpret identical actions and outcomes in radically different ways depending on the motives and intentions underlying them. Moreover, we take reckoning of ourselves stacked up against others, and ideally make moral decisions with others in mind. Recently, evidence has been accumulating suggesting that our closest relatives are also sensitive to the motives of others and can distinguish intentional from accidental actions. These results suggest that chimpanzees interpret the actions of others from a psychological perspective, not just a behavioural perspective. However, based on recent studies, it is not clear whether chimpanzees have any regard *for* others, calling into the question the point at which fairness and other-regard were used as building blocks for full-fledged human morality.

2006 Empathy and Fairness. Wiley, Chichester (Novartis Foundation Symposium 278) p 56–70

If I spill coffee on your shirt, you are likely to view my action in a very different light depending on whether I did this by accident or on purpose. In the first case, you may consider me clumsy, and perhaps after the initial shock had waned, even feel pity for my clumsiness. In the second case your attitude toward me will be totally different. You may consider me a person with a warped sense of humour at best, even a nasty and unfair person in the worst case. The remarkable thing is that in both cases my action produced the same outcome and what distinguishes them is the psychological motive underlying it. In effect, reading and taking into account the motives and intentions of others is a fundamental part of human social interaction. Often actions and outcomes are not so important, it is the motive behind them that really matters.

Numerous developmental psychologists have suggested that the beginnings of such special human sensitivity to the psychological states of others underlying actions can already be seen in very young infants (e.g. Bertenthal 1996, Carpenter et al 1998, D'Entremont et al 1997, Meltzoff 1995). Much less is known about how non-human animals, including our closest relatives, interpret the actions of others. Are non-human animals restricted to the observable behaviour of others in social interaction or do they also show some sensitivity to the motives of others? In this chapter we will tackle this question from two complementary directions. First, we will review recent studies on the understanding of intentional actions in apes, more specifically regarding the distinction between intentional and accidental actions. Second, we will review recent studies about whether individuals are self- or other-regarding. We chose to focus on these two areas because they appear to be key components in the evolution of fairness and morality. In the final section of the chapter, we will briefly speculate about the implications of this research for the evolution of fairness and morality in nonhuman animals and highlight future research directions.

Distinguishing intentional from accidental actions

Understanding intentional action in others is a skill that allows human infants to parse the complex streams of behaviour displayed by adults (Baldwin et al 2001). By being attuned to the intentions and goals of others, infants can anticipate the behaviour of others, can learn from others (even in the absence of the solution), and can explain the behaviour of others more effectively. Given such a central role in the development of social cognition, it is not surprising that the study of intentional and goal-directed action has received considerable attention in recent years. By 6 months of age, infants have expectations about human actions, but not about inanimate objects performing similar actions. Woodward (1999) interpreted these results as evidence that infants perceive actions as goal directed. By 9 months of age infants can distinguish the motives behind certain actions (Behne et al 2005), understand the actions of entities as goal-directed, and expect the use of efficient actions to achieve those goals (Gergely & Csibra 2003, Gergely et al 1995). Starting at 14 months of age infants can distinguish accidental versus intentional actions (Carpenter et al 1998), perceive that others choose plans of action that meet the requirements of the situation (Gergely et al 2002), and can use unfulfilled actions on objects to produce the intended goal of a demonstrator (Meltzoff 1995).

Although Premack & Woodruff's (1978) study on chimpanzee intentions signalled the starting point for the now vast literature on children's theory of mind, comparatively little progress has been made with non-human animals since then. There are only a handful of studies devoted to the study of goals and intentions—and these represent a patchy collection of positive, negative and unclear results. Here, we will concentrate on those paradigms that have produced data both for children and apes and that have investigated whether individuals perceive the distinction between intentional and accidental actions in others (see Call 2005, Call & Tomasello 2005, Tomasello & Call 2006, for a broader coverage on this topic).

Call & Tomasello (1998) trained chimpanzees and orangutans to use a landmark placed on top of one of three opaque containers as an indicator for the location of hidden food. During training the apes never saw the human actually placing the marker on the container, but the marker was already on top of one of the containers when they were presented to the ape. On test trials a human experimenter then placed the marker on one of the containers intentionally, but either before or after this he let the marker fall accidentally onto one of the other containers. The marker was removed at the time of choice of the ape, so for test trials the ape was faced with a choice in which one bucket had been marked with the marker intentionally and the other accidentally. Apes as a group chose the container that was marked intentionally, although no individual except a language-trained orangutan was above chance on his own. The apes' performance was comparable to that of 2.5-year-old children presented with the same task and worse than that of 3-year-old children. In contrast, we found no evidence that dogs tested with the same paradigm distinguished between intentional and accidental actions (Riedel et al 2006).

There are some neurological data that support the idea that primates do indeed perceive the distinction between intentional and accidental actions. Jellema et al (2000) have described a population of cells in the superior temporal sulcus (STS) of the macaque that respond to the orientation of the face in combination with actions. Those same neurons do not respond if those same actions are performed while the subject's attention is focused elsewhere. Recall that in the previous experiment, the focus of attention was one of the main indicators of intention. Intentional actions were those that are attended to whereas accidental actions invariably occurred when the attention was averted from the action.

We used another paradigm to investigate whether chimpanzees can gauge the motives of a human experimenter (Call et al 2004). More specifically, we tested whether in a food-sharing situation they can distinguish between a human who is unwilling to give them food from one who is unable to do so. Thus, we presented chimpanzees with a situation in which a human gave them food through a hole in their cage (see Fig. 1). After the experimenter had passed a few grapes to the subject, he took another grape but did not pass it to the subject and we manipulated the reasons for stopping the transfer. In some cases, he was unable because the hole was too small, he was occupied with other tasks, or he did not see the food. In other cases, he was unwilling to give the food. In such trials he put the food close to the ape but then pulled it back, or left the food on the platform and stared at the ape for no apparent reason, or just ate the food. Overall, we presented three trios of unwilling and unable conditions. Each trio consisted of an unwilling condition paired with two unable conditions. Each trio shared some basic features such as the overall motions of the grape or the experimenter's gazing pattern.

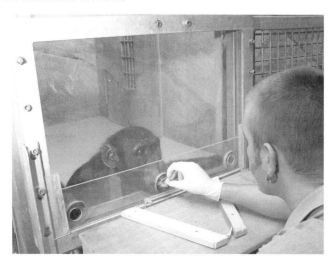

FIG. 1. Testing situation for the unwilling–unable experiment.

The reason for having multiple conditions organized in trios was double. First, we wanted to get as many conditions as possible so that a potential difference could not be accounted by a superficial difference between a single unwilling and a single unable condition. Second, organizing the conditions by trios allowed us to control to some extent the effect some variables such as the reward's motion patterns and the eye contact between the experimenter and the subject. For instance, if we only had a single unwilling condition that involved eye contact between the experimenter and the subject and a single unable condition that did not, then one could argue that any differences between conditions was due to the presence of eye contact. Eye contact may have simply made subjects more nervous and that, not intention assessment, was the reason underlying the observed differences.

Some important methodological considerations of this study are that we did not train subjects to respond in any way, they were not differentially reinforced for their responses, and we only administered two trials per condition. Instead we scored the natural reactions of the chimpanzees and assessed whether they behaved differentially across conditions. In particular we scored two variables: behaviours directed at the experimenter or the food (in most cases these were aimed at convincing the experimenter to transfer the food) and how long subjects remained at the testing station without receiving food. Chimpanzees reacted in different ways to unwilling and unable conditions. When the experimenter was unwilling, they gestured more and they left the testing station earlier than when the experimenter was unable to pass the food. This difference existed even though they were not differentially rewarded. One can postulate a different explanation for each difference across conditions or one can argue that the underlying principal is behind several of those conditions. Behne et al (2005) found comparable findings with 9- to 18-month-old human infants, but not with 6-month-olds.

In summary, chimpanzees distinguished between an experimenter who was unwilling from one who was unable to give them food. They also distinguished the intentional from the accidental actions of a human in a communicative situation. Thus, these results suggest that apes may go beyond the observable information and infer the goals of others in particular situations.

Regard for others

Until now we have presented some evidence suggesting that apes, like humans, can distinguish intentional from accidental actions. This, combined with data recently gathered on perspective taking (see Tomasello & Call 2006 for a review), suggests that chimpanzees, at least, may interpret the actions of others from a psychological perspective (Tomasello et al 2003, but see Povinelli & Vonk 2003). Such sophistication can have important repercussions in the way these species appraise their interactions with others. While they might regard others as intentional agents, do apes and other nonhuman animals use this information to guide their behaviours? Are they other-regarding; do they care for fairness? We turn now to the second area in our review.

It is hard to imagine someone with regard for others who does not recognize that the individuals he is harming or helping are, like him, capable of suffering and experiencing pleasure. Presumably, if the actor recognizes others as having intentions, he can recognize that they can be frustrated if their goals are not met. Furthermore, he should care. On the simplest level, an other-regarding individual should be able to compare his goals and the degree to which they are met with the goals and outcomes of other individuals. Humans are notorious for social comparison—it is not enough to have a big TV if the Joneses have a bigger one. Our sense of social comparison, of other-regard, is not always positive. Our sensitivity to fairness is biased toward ourselves, what Fehr & Schmidt (1999) call disadvantageous inequity aversion.

To prevent unfairness, individuals should try, at the very least, to avoid or prevent situations that put themselves at a disadvantage relative to others. It seems most likely that this kind of comparative selfishness would be the bare minimum for other-regard. If an individual acts to prevent an unfair outcome, even at a cost to himself with no direct benefit, then this individual is spiteful. Spite seems to be the force that drives people to reject unfair offers in the ultimatum game; people who reject unfair offers tend to be angry (Pillutla & Murnighan 1996). Altruistic punishment is the term sometimes used for this costly reaction to inequities (Fehr & Gächter 2002, Boyd et al 2003), and forms the basis for strong reciprocity

(Gintis et al 2003). Whether the motivation is ultimately altruistic or not, the situation that provokes the punishment is unfairness.

Brosnan & de Waal (2003) were the first to address the question of unfairness in non-human primates, namely capuchins (*Cebus apella*) and chimpanzees (Brosnan et al 2005). They found that capuchins and chimpanzees (though to a far smaller degree), reject unfair food offers from an experimenter. However, one of the problems with these studies is that rejecting an unfair offer actually increases inequity. The animals were powerless to correct inequitable situations. Brosnan, now teamed up with Silk and others (Silk et al 2005), gave a task to chimpanzees where they could bring food toward themselves, while at the same time providing food for non-kin conspecifics. What they found was that chimpanzees sometimes chose selfishly so that only they got the food for their efforts, and just as often they chose mutualistically so that the free-rider also benefited. In other words, the chimpanzees appeared indifferent to the outcome of their actions on another chimpanzee.

We used a similar logic in a series of three experiments (Jensen et al 2006, see Fig. 2). In the first, captive chimpanzees could pull a table with food toward herself, so that she alone could access a quarter of a banana (selfishness), or toward herself and a male group member (either the alpha male or a five-year old male; mutualism). Chimpanzees were strongly mutualistic. Or so it would seem. But in a control condition, they showed precisely the same preference when the room was empty. It is not clear from this study whether chimpanzees were intentionally mutualistic, but it is clear that they were not sensitive to unfairness (because, after all, the males got to eat the same amount of food without sharing in any of the work).

In the second study, the chimpanzees could pull food toward the same males as before, or toward an inaccessible area. The former choice would be altruistic and the latter would be spiteful because the recipient's banana would be pulled further away. In no case could the actor get a banana. Half the time, the chimpanzees did nothing, which meant that the recipients got nothing. The remainder of the time they were as likely to pull food toward the recipient as to pull the opposite table. Now it could be that the chimpanzees, by doing nothing, were being passively spiteful, and combined with their truly spiteful choices, were demonstrating a clear aversion to disadvantageous inequity by depriving the other chimpanzee of food more than three-quarters of the time.

However, in the third study, the table holding a banana piece for the waiting recipient moved toward him on its own in a 'ghost pull,' and chimpanzees did nothing even more often, leading to the recipient getting the banana roughly 90% of the time. (There was now no banana piece on the inaccessible table since it seemed that chimpanzees often pulled that one in the previous study with the unfulfilled goal of making the banana fly within their own reach.) This 'passive

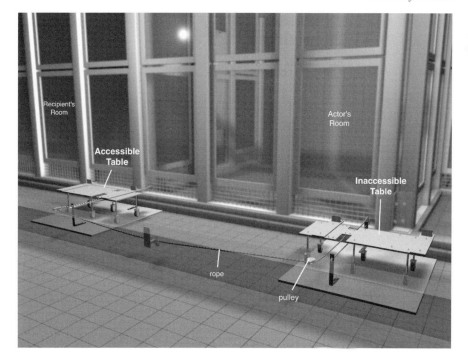

FIG. 2.   Testing apparatus and set-up for the self-regard studies. Two tables sit outside of the
chimpanzees' reach, and only the one in the middle can pull them closer. Because they are
connected, pulling one table closer causes the other to move further away. If the actor pulls
the table to her right (accessible table), the choice is either mutualistic (both get food) or altruistic (only the recipient gets food). If the actor pulls the inaccessible table to her left, she is
either being selfish (eats alone) or spiteful (prevents the recipient from getting food). (Reproduced from Proc R Soc B; Jensen et al 2006.)

altruism' contradicts any 'passive spite' argument from the previous study, and
shows that chimpanzees were merely passive; they were indifferent to the outcomes for the others. Interestingly, two chimpanzees showed a tendency toward
altruism when the spite stakes were higher. One pulled food toward both males,
then quietly—and fruitlessly—begged from them. The other pulled food only
toward the low-ranking male and then threatened him. It is questionable how
altruistic their motives were.

The results of these three studies, as well as those of Silk et al (2005), contradict
earlier claims of inequity aversion in chimpanzees. Further studies will be needed
to determine whether or not chimpanzees and other non-human animals are sensitive to outcomes that affect others. That chimpanzees—or any species at all—are
self-regarding is no surprise. It is somewhat surprising to consider that the com-

parison of relative costs and benefits may be uniquely human. In the absence of other-regard, crucial features for cooperation and morality may be relatively recent evolutionary products exhibited only by humans. Or it may be that other-regard in other species works in some contexts but not others.

Social interaction, intentions and the evolution of morality

The final question of our contribution is what impact these findings may have on the debate on fairness and morality in non-human animals. Although we know that perceiving others' intentions shapes the way humans classify others as good or evil, we have to admit that we know relatively little about this aspect in non-human animals. The data available in chimpanzees suggest that although they distinguish intentional from accidental actions in others, they show little evidence of other-regard. This contrast is perhaps even more puzzling if one considers that chimpanzees are capable of image scoring, that is, they prefer to beg food from a human who has shared food with others compared to one who has refused to do so (Russell et al 2006).

One possibility is that although chimpanzees can determine who is willing, unwilling, or unable to share food with them both through direct as well as indirect interactions (i.e. observed), such distinctions still fall short of abstracting certain attitudinal qualities of individuals. For instance, do chimpanzees that are sensitive to whether someone is willing or not to give them food also classify them as dependable or non-dependable, and more importantly, do they use this knowledge in future interactions with them? We do not know the answer to this question. Only additional research will be able to tell us.

One important aspect of human attribution in helping situations is that they often carry a moral judgment. The person that does not share when nothing prevents her from doing so is not only seen as unwilling, she is also seen as wicked and unfair. In fact, for humans evaluating a situation in which somebody did not offer help because she was unable to see the person requesting help or because she was unable to offer help because her access was blocked are important pieces of information. And such information determines the moral judgment. It is conceivable that apes may perceive the first part (the unwilling part) but perhaps do not take the next step (the unfair part). The person that does not share food, may not be seen as unfair; it is simply a person that it is not willing to share food, an instrumental rather than a moral appraisal. Whether moral judgments are attached to certain actions in non-human animals is something that again deserves further scrutiny.

In conclusion, chimpanzees distinguish intentional from accidental actions, can eavesdrop information by observing the interactions of third parties, but there is little evidence that they are other-regarding. Whether apes dress their interpretations of actions with a moralistic layer (good vs. evil, fair vs. unfair) remains unclear and further research is needed.

References

Baldwin DA, Baird JA, Saylor MM, Clark MA 2001 Infants parse dynamic action. Child Dev 72:708–717

Behne T, Carpenter M, Call J, Tomasello M 2005 Unwilling or unable? Infants' understanding of others' intentions. Dev Psychol 41:328–337

Bertenthal B 1996 Origins and early development of perception, action, and representation. Annu Rev Psychol 47:431–59

Boyd R, Gintis H, Bowles S, Richerson PJ 2003 The evolution of altruistic punishment. Proc Natl Acad Sci 100:3531–3535

Brosnan S, de Waal FBM 2003 Monkeys reject unequal pay. Nature 425:297–299

Brosnan SF, Schiff HC, de Waal FBM 2005 Tolerance for inequity may increase with social closeness in chimpanzees. Proc R Soc Biol Sci Ser B 272:253–258

Call J 2005 Chimpanzees are sensitive to some of the psychological states of others. Interaction Studies 6:413–427

Call J, Tomasello M 1998 Distinguishing intentional from accidental actions in orangutans (*Pongo pygmaeus*), chimpanzees (*Pan troglodytes*) and human children (*Homo sapiens*). J Comp Psychol 112:192–206

Call J, Tomasello M 2005 What chimpanzees know about seeing revisited: An explanation of the third kind. In: Eilan N, Hoerl C, McCormack T, Roessler J (eds) Joint attention: communication and other minds. Oxford University Press, Oxford, p 45–64

Call J, Hare B, Carpenter M, Tomasello M 2004 Unwilling or unable: Chimpanzees' understanding of human intentional action. Developmental Sci 7:488–498

Carpenter M, Akhtar N, Tomasello M 1998 Fourteen- through 18-month-old infants differentially imitate intentional and accidental actions. Infant Behav Dev 21:315–330

D'Entremont B, Hains SMJ, Muir DW 1997 A demonstration of gaze following in 3- to 6-month-olds. Infant Behav & Dev 20:569–572

Fehr E, Schmidt KM 1999 A theory of fairness, competition, and cooperation. Q J Econom 114:817–868

Fehr E, Gächter S 2002 Altruistic punishment in humans. Nature 415:137–140

Gergely G, Csibra G 2003 Teleological reasoning in infancy: the naïve theory of rational action. Trends Cogn Sci 7:287–292

Gergely G, Nádasdy Z, Csibra G, Bíró S 1995 Taking the intentional stance at 12 months of age. Cognition 56:165–193

Gergely G, Bekkering H, Király I 2002 Rational imitation in preverbal infants. Nature 415:755

Gintis H, Bowles S, Boyd R, Fehr E 2003 Explaining altruistic behavior in humans. Evol Hum Behav 24:153–172

Jellema T, Baker CI, Wicker B, Perrett DI 2000 Neural representation for the perception of the intentionality of actions. Brain Cogn 44:280–302

Jensen K, Hare B, Call J, Tomasello M 2006 What's in it for me? Self-regard precludes altruism and spite in chimpanzees. Proc R Soc Biol Sci Ser B 273:1013–1021

Meltzoff A 1995 Understanding the intentions of others: Re-enactment of intended acts by 18-month-old children. Dev Psychol 31:1–16

Pillutla M, Murnighan J 1996 Unfairness, anger, and spite: emotional rejections of ultimatum offers. Organ Behav Hum Decis Process 68:208–224

Povinelli DJ, Vonk J 2003 Chimpanzee minds: Suspiciously human? Trends Cogn Sci 7:157–160

Premack D, Woodruff G 1978 Does the chimpanzee have a theory of mind? Behav Brain Sci Behav 4:51–526

Riedel J, Buttlemann D, Call J, Tomasello M 2006 Domestic dogs (Canis familiaris) use a physical marker to locate hidden food. Anim Cogn 9:27–35

Russell YI, Call J, Dunbar RIM 2006 Image scoring in great apes. Submitted

Silk JB, Brosnan SF, Vonk J et al 2005 Chimpanzees are indifferent to the welfare of unrelated group members. Nature 437:1357–1359

Tomasello M, Call J 2006 Do chimpanzees know what others see—or only what they are looking at? In: Hurley S, Nudds M (eds) Rational animals. Oxford University Press, Oxford p371–384

Tomasello M, Call J, Hare B 2003 Chimpanzees understand psychological states—the question is which ones and to what extent. Trends Cogn Sci 7:153–156

Woodward A 1999 Infants' ability to distinguish between purposeful and non-purposeful behaviors. Infant Behav Dev 22:145–160

DISCUSSION

Silk: We have done experiments similar to one of your experiments which provided the chimps with an opportunity to provide rewards to others at no cost to themselves, with chimps at two different facilities in the USA, and got exactly the same results (Silk et al 2005). The studies are eerily similar.

Hauser: I want to ask about your experiment involving different responses to different partners. It is not clear to me yet that you can say anything yet about reputation from these data. Let's say that for the last 20 times when there has been an opportunity for you and I to cooperate, you have cooperated. All of a sudden you cheat. I am probably going to label you a cheater. But if you had cheated 20 times and cooperated once, I am not going to convert you to being a cooperator. There seems to be a strong asymmetry here. If you saw a subject have repeated experiences with the same individual where there was a run of one interaction and then an exception, would the subject change behaviour or stick to the pattern? It seems to me you don't need to go with the slapping; just not giving the food would seem to be enough.

Call: The reason for the slapping is that we wanted the extreme. Once we get that, then we can do variations such as those you suggested.

Hauser: Then you could understand how they actually do build a reputation, and how many repeats are needed.

Call: Another addition would be to see what happens when you put the same people in a different game. Will they be treated differently?

Brosnan: I had a question about that experiment too. It is odd that they became more likely to choose the nice guy over time, rather than less likely. Based on my experience with chimps, I would have expected that by the fourth trial they wouldn't even pay attention to you any more since they weren't getting any food. Do you have any speculations on why this might be?

Call: They did! They get food at the end of each trial from the keeper. They don't get food from the nice and nasty guys. This is just four trials done on four different days. It is interesting to look at the individual differences. Who are the guys that approach and those who don't? This is something we need to look into.

Brosnan: In the four trials is the same person always the nice one?

Call: Yes.

Brosnan: Perhaps the slap is at least starting to attract their attention and they think if they do it differently they will get some food.

Call: We could look at their reactions over time to see whether they get used to the slapping? The reaction was quite strong initially, but we haven't looked over time.

Dupoux: In the first experiment, the one you called direct reputation, it looks as if the chimps are trying to assess the probability of getting food. When the subject is unable to give them the food they may think there is a possibility that it may get through some way or another. This is far from being a reputation.

Call: I am not tied to the word 'reputation'. I would say that this is the first stepping stone towards something that could be reputation. If you can see this across a number of different studies and the same people are treated differentially across studies, then I would call this direct reputation. This refers here to information gained by direct interaction as opposed to information gained through observing the interaction of third parties.

Dupoux: In the second study the nasty person is actually both inflicting pain and not cooperating. It would be nice to disentangle these.

Singer: Could you add trust and reciprocity games, as we use them in humans, to your experiment after your manipulation of reputation formation in chimps? Could chimps in principle understand that if they give you one banana they will always get three times as much in return?

Call: They could play this game with a human, but between two chimps it would be hard.

Singer: Would the chimpanzee understand the concept of giving one banana and getting three in exchange?

Call: There are studies on delay of gratification in chimps where they will not eat one banana now but rather wait to get three.

Singer: Then you could add such games as a second phase to the reputation formation study and see whether chimps would trust people more with good rather than bad reputations.

Call: Sarah Brosnan has done some studies with humans distributing food between two chimps.

Sigman: Does your group have data on children in experiments like this?

Call: Keith Jensen is starting this with children but the data collection is not completed. There is more altruism in children than chimpanzees.

Silk: I know one study that we discovered after we did our experiments (Thompson et al 1997). This is a study of 3–5 year old children in which they are offered a choice between one sticker for themselves and one for the experimenter (a friendly female), or one sticker for themselves. Between the ages of 3 and 5 there are no age effects, but 85% of the children choose the choice that gives one sticker to themselves and one to the experimenter. If you offer the choice of two for the child and none for the experimenter, about 65% of children still want a sticker for themselves and one for the experimenter. We are starting some work on children using food rewards.

Dupoux: We are also doing these sorts of experiments.

Spinrad: Nancy Eisenberg and her colleagues have differentiated between spontaneous sharing and compliant sharing (Eisenberg et al 1981, Eisenberg-Berg & Hand 1979, see Eisenberg & Fabes 1998). You are examining more compliant forms of sharing; do you have any intention of investigating more spontaneous sharing, perhaps in the same type of paradigm?

Call: What would you predict?

Spinrad: Spontaneous sharing would have a higher cost, so we would view this type of sharing as more altruistic. In some of Nancy's work, preschoolers' spontaneous sharing was positively related to higher level, rudimentary needs-oriented moral reasoning (Eisenberg et al 1984, Eisenberg-Berg & Hand 1979), whereas preschoolers who were high in compliant sharing/prosocial behaviours appeared to be non-assertive (Eisenberg et al 1981, 1990, 1984).

Hauser: There is also some work by Jeff Stevens on harassment being a prod to cooperation (Stevens 2004) in squirrel monkeys and chimpanzees. This appears to be a cost-free mechanism to get cooperation going without punishment.

Call: In the mid-1970s Richard Wrangham published his food sharing hypothesis (Wrangham 1975). When you look at the chimpanzee food sharing, a lot of it takes place under pressure. I don't think this hypothesis is getting the attention it deserves.

Van Lange: There is a nice link between these results and the noise in social interaction, 'noise' meaning that there are unintended effects. The recipient doesn't know whether there was an intentional benefit, or whether it was just an accident. There is often noise in everyday systems. This might be a nice direction to go in when we look at ability versus willingness. Sometimes the other ape doesn't know whether an act is intentional.

Call: One of the conditions in the first study is that we tried to put the food through but then it fell. It was an accident. When we look at this condition it seems different from the teasing one. Some actions in that study are accidental; others involve some physical blockage that prevents us from passing the food. We deliberately tried different actions because we wanted to make sure it wasn't just about teasing and something else. We wanted to test how generalizable these responses were.

Gallese: There are two conflicting intentions which are readily recognized by the animal. In one case it looks like I intend to give the food, then all of a sudden I withdraw it. Then in the other case I keep on pushing, so there is just one intention, that of giving the food, but some local constraint prevents this.

Call: That is true. The other component of that trio of experiments involved dropping grapes as they are about to be put through the hole. The grape rolls down and you pick it up again. This is like the teasing experiment.

C Frith: I am very struck by your result showing a strong distinction between an intentional and an unintentional action. The chimpanzees can recognize this. It seemed to have a powerful effect in Tanya Singer's experiment, too: you only dislike the person when what they are doing is volitional. This suggests that this is an important distinction. To what extent does this also apply in the moral dilemmas that Mark Hauser described? He described one where there was an asymmetry between good and harm. We weren't convinced this is actually what is taking place. The assistant comes in and says they have a new process that will make more profit but it will also harm the environment. At that stage the director has to make a decision between profit and environment. In another situation the assistant says there is a new process that will make more profit and help the environment. In this case no choice has to be made because there is no conflict—since there was no choice the director is not seen as responsible. But there is another scenario: if the assistant says that the new process will help the environment but will make less profit. In this case, if the director says they will adopt this process, people will say he was responsible for this. Deciding whether or not someone is responsible for their actions is a crucial aspect of how we understand other people and how we respond to them.

Hauser: In both cases the CEO says 'I don't care about helping or harming, all I care about is making money'. What comes up as a side-effect is irrelevant because their intention is only to make money. Then someone asks the question, did she or he intend for the side-effect to happen?

C Frith: What I am suggesting is that it doesn't really matter whether the side-effect is good or bad: the critical thing is whether he or she has to make a real decision.

Hauser: The CEO is making a decision about the policy in terms of its money-making. There is an asymmetry in what is being attributed. He is saying he doesn't care about the consequences.

Moll: What if you change the situation as follows: you say there is a procedure that involves the installation of certain equipment, incurring in certain costs, but which will help the environment. The question would then be to install it or not.

Hauser: There we find the action/omission bias coming in strongly. We see this even in four year old children. In one scenario, Billy does not like his sister Susie. Susie is going to a birthday party and lays out her favourite dress. Billy takes her dress and puts it outside during a rainstorm so that it gets ruined. That is case one. In case two, Billy doesn't like his sister, it starts to rain, and Billy leaves her dress outside so it gets wet. There is the same consequence and same intention, but children quickly say that Billy in the first case was worse than in the second case. It is the action/omission bias which is there early on and strongly.

Frank: The history of the distinction may turn on how easy it is to infer intention in the two cases. You can construct hypothetical examples in which the intention was the same in each, but in practice we don't often encounter situations knowing what someone's intention was.

Hauser: This is relevant to some of the earlier discussions about the animal work on deception. Omissions were easy for people to uncover, but commissions were quite hard to find.

Moll: You classify a person as a cheater, attributing a reputation code. This concept about the person can then help you make inferences. It can bias inferences. If you know that this person is capable of doing something, you are more likely to infer that specific intentional state, using a simple heuristic strategy.

Gergely: What is the basis of the choice between nice and nasty that the chimps make? Do they see one as a source of food and the other not? You could combine the able and unable paradigms, with having two guys where the chimp would get three pieces of food from both of them, but one of them would drop it in a way that looked accidental.

Call: Yes, we could combine the first study and second study and see the distinctions they make when they are interacting one-to-one with a human. If they see a teaser and non-teaser interacting, it would be interesting to see whether they prefer to take food from the non-teaser.

Silk: Have you thought of taking the videos from these experiments and letting the chimps watch them? You could then ask whether chimpanzees pay attention to how others behave in these kinds of situations, and if they will then make use of that reputational information in their own interactions with potential partners.

Call: We want to start using video. We want to start with social learning to see whether we get them watching. If they do, we can then do some manipulations.

Brosnan: Have you seen Sarah Poss' work (Poss & Rochat 2003)? For her dissertation, she looked at whether chimpanzees attend to video. She had two tubes that were different colours, and in one she put peanut butter. They watched a video of her doing this. She then offered the tubes to the chimps, who had one choice and received the tube they choose. They did just as well picking the tube containing peanut butter watching the video as they did after seeing her fill the tube in front of them.

Frank: Had they seen her doing this task before they watched the video?

Brosnan: I don't remember.

References

Eisenberg-Berg N, Hand M 1979 The relationship of preschooler's reasoning about prosocial moral conflicts to prosocial behavior. Child Dev 50:356–363

Eisenberg N, Fabes R 1998 Prosocial development. In: Damon W, Eisenberg N (eds), Handbook of child psychology, vol 3: Social, emotional, and personality development (5th ed). Wiley, New York, p 701–778

Eisenberg N, Cameron E, Tryon K, Dodez R 1981 Socialization of prosocial behavior in the preschool classroom. Dev Psychol 17:773–782

Eisenberg N, Fabes RA, Miller PA, Shell C, Shea R, May-Plumlee T 1990 Preschoolers' vicarious emotional responding and their situational and dispositional prosocial behavior. Merrill-Palmer Quarterly 36:507–529

Eisenberg N, Fabes RA, Murphy B et al 1994 The relations of emotionality and regulation to dispositional and situational empathy-related responding. J Personal Social Psychol 66:776–797

Poss S, Rochat P 2003 Referential understanding of videos in chimpanzees (*Pan troglodytes*), orangutans, (*Pongo pygmaeus*), and children (*Homo sapiens*). J Comp Psychol 117:420–428

Silk JB, Brosnan SF, Vonk J et al 2005 Chimpanzees are indifferent to the welfare of unrelated group members. Nature 437:1357–1359

Stevens JR 2004 The selfish nature of generosity: harassment and food sharing in primates. Proc Roy Soc Lond B 271:451–456

Thompson C, Barresi J, Moore C 1997 The development of future-oriented prudence and altruism in preschoolers. Cognit Devel 12:199–212

Wrangham R 1975 The behavioural ecology of chimpanzee in Gombe National Park, Tanzania. PhD thesis, Cambridge University

Empathy-related responding and prosocial behaviour

Nancy Eisenberg[1]

Department of Psychology, Box 871104, Tempe, AZ 85287–1104, USA

Abstract. In this paper I differentiate among empathy, sympathy and personal distress and discuss the central role of empathy-related responding in positive (including moral) development. Empathy-related responding, especially sympathy, is likely an important source of prosocial, other-oriented motivation. In fact, empathy-related responding, especially sympathy, has been associated with prosocial behaviour (voluntary behaviour intended to benefit another, e.g. helping, sharing); this relation has been obtained for both specific instances of empathy-related responding and for dispositional sympathy. In addition, sympathy (or sometimes empathy) has been linked to relatively high levels of moral reasoning and social competence, and to low levels of aggression and antisocial behaviour. In my talk, I will review research on the relation of empathy-related responding to prosocial behaviour, the consistency of costly prosocial behaviour over time and the possible role of sympathy in its consistency, and the relation of empathy-related responding to moral reasoning, antisocial behaviour and social competence. Examples of research, including longitudinal research in our laboratory, are provided to illustrate these relations. Because of its close relations to social and prosocial responding, an understanding of empathy-related responding contributes to efforts to promote children's moral development.

2006 Empathy and Fairness. Wiley, Chichester (Novartis Foundation Symposium 278) p 71–96

In recent decades numerous psychologists have proposed that empathy-related responding, including caring or sympathetic concern, motivates moral behaviour, especially prosocial behaviour, inhibits aggression and other antisocial behaviours, and contributes to the broader domain of social competence (Eisenberg & Fabes 1998, Hoffman 2000). Thus, psychologists have increasingly recognized the potential importance of empathy-related responding in moral and social development.

Despite strong conceptual reasons to expect a relationship between empathy and prosocial behaviour, in 1982 Underwood and Moore published a review in which they found, contrary to most theory, *no* empirical relation between empathy

---

[1]Unfortunately, Nancy Eisenberg was unable to attend the symposium. In her absence, this paper was presented by her colleague, Tracy Spinrad.

and prosocial behaviour such as helping and sharing (Underwood & Moore 1982). However, most of the work before 1982 had been conducted with children using measures that were problematic and there were conceptual problems with most of the existing research.

Conceptual Issues

In regard to the conceptual limitations in the work, most investigators had not differentiated between different types of empathy-related responding that would be expected to involve different affective motivations. Batson (1991) first differentiated between empathy and personal distress in the late 1970s. Making yet one more distinction (between empathy and sympathy), we define *empathy* as an affective response that stems from the apprehension or comprehension of another's emotional state or condition, and which is similar to what the other person is feeling or would be expected to feel. Thus, if someone views a sad person and consequently feels sad him or herself, that person is experiencing empathy.

In most situations, especially after infancy or when the empathy is more than fleeting, empathy is likely to evolve into sympathy, personal distress, or both. *Sympathy* is defined as an emotional response stemming from the apprehension of another's emotional state or condition that is not the same as the other's state or condition, but consists of feelings of sorrow or concern for the other. Thus, if a boy sees a distressed peer and feels concern for the peer, he is experiencing sympathy. It is probable that sympathy is often based upon empathic sadness, although it also may be experienced as a consequence of cognitive perspective taking or accessing information from memory that is relevant to the other's experience (Eisenberg 1986).

Empathy can also lead to personal distress. *Personal distress* is a self-focused, aversive affective reaction to the apprehension of another's emotion (e.g. discomfort, anxiety). As for sympathy, personal distress sometimes may stem from empathy if the empathic response is experienced as too arousing and as aversive. However, it is also possible that personal distress sometimes stems from other emotion-related processes (e.g. guilt) or from retrieving certain information from mental storage.

It is also important to differentiate between prosocial behaviour and altruism. *Prosocial behaviour* is defined as voluntary behaviour intended to benefit another (e.g. helping, sharing and comforting). Prosocial behaviours can be motivated by a variety of factors, including egoistic concerns (rewards or social approval), other-oriented concern (e.g. sympathy), or moral values (e.g. the desire to uphold internalized moral values). *Altruistic behaviour* often is defined as those prosocial behaviours motivated by other-oriented or moral concerns/emotion rather than concrete or social rewards or the desire to reduce one's own aversive affective states (Eisenberg 1986).

These conceptual nuances are critical when attempting to predict prosocial behaviour or other outcomes from empathy-related responding. For example, sympathy and personal distress are expected to result in different motivations and, consequently, different behaviour. Batson (1991) proposed that a sympathetic emotional reaction (labelled empathy by Batson) is associated with the desire to reduce the other person's distress or need and therefore is likely to lead to altruistic behaviour if the cost is not too high. In contrast, personal distress, because it is an aversive experience, is believed to be associated with the motivation to reduce one's own distress and the desire to avoid contact with the needy or distressed other if possible. People experiencing personal distress would be expected to assist only when helping is the easiest way to reduce the helper's own distress.

Empirical Issues

In regard to methodological issues, most of the early studies on children's empathy involved the use of picture-story measures of empathy, in which children were told a number of very short stories about evocative events (e.g. a child who lost his/her dog or at a birthday party), accompanied by a small number of illustrations. After hearing each story, children were asked how they themselves felt. It is doubtful that these stories elicited much emotion, yet children were asked how they felt and often may have responded based on social desirability concerns. Indeed, performance on these measures was at best weakly related to prosocial behaviour and was influenced heavily by factors such as sex of the experimenter (see Eisenberg & Miller 1987).

Thus, there was a need for better measures of empathy-related responding. The experimental methods and self-report measures Batson (1991) used were in general inappropriate for use with children. Consequently, Richard Fabes and I conducted a series of studies designed to validate alternative measures of empathy-related responding and to examine their relations to children's prosocial behaviour.

Specifically, we used self-report, facial, and physiological markers of sympathy and personal distress. In a first set of studies, we found that when children or adults were in situations likely to induce a reaction akin to personal distress (e.g. in response to a film), they exhibited higher heart rate (HR) and skin conductance (SC) than in analogous situations that were likely to induce sympathy. We suggested that HR acceleration might reflect distress whereas HR deceleration reflects interest in, and processing of information, coming from external stimuli, in this case, the sympathy-inducing stimulus. Moreover, children and adults tended to exhibit facial concerned attention rather than distress in sympathy-inducing contexts, and older children's and adults' self-reports also were somewhat consistent with the emotional context (see Eisenberg & Fabes 1990, 1998, Eisenberg et al 1991a).

Next, in another set of studies we examined the relation of our measures of sympathetic or personal distress reactions during empathy-inducing films about others to helping or sharing with the needy and/or distressed individuals in the film (or others like them) when it was easy to avoid contact with them. For example, children would view a film of a child who was injured and in the hospital and was talking about the experience. We would measure heart rate and/or skin conductance while the children watched the film, taped and coded their facial reactions to the film, and, after the film, asked them to rate how they felt during the film. A short time later, they had the opportunity to assist the person(s) in the film or similar others by doing donating earnings or time or doing a boring task to help the children rather than playing with attractive toys. Consistent with expectations, markers of sympathy generally were positively related to prosocial behaviour whereas markers of personal distress were negatively related to prosocial behaviour, the latter particularly for children. Thus, sympathy and personal distress seemed to reflect quite different motivational states (Eisenberg & Fabes 1990, 1998).

The relation of empathy-related responding to the long term prediction of prosocial dispositions

In our work on prosocial behaviour, we have found that there is considerable consistency over time in the types of prosocial behaviours that are likely to be other-oriented in origin and that sympathy or empathy may play a role in this consistency. We have conducted a 25 year study of prosocial moral reasoning and prosocial responding. When the children were 4–5 years old, their naturally occurring prosocial behaviours were observed in the preschool classroom for months and were coded as occurring spontaneously (without a peer's verbal or non-verbal request) or in response to a request (compliant), and as helping or sharing (little comforting was observed). Helping behaviours generally were low in cost, such as tying a peer's apron. Sharing was higher cost because it required giving up of an object or space in the child's possession. We found that spontaneous sharing, but not the other types of prosocial behaviour, was related to children's references to others' needs in the assessment of their prosocial moral reasoning. Thus, children's other-oriented concerns when reasoning about hypothetical moral dilemmas—probably based on rudimentary perspective taking and empathy/sympathy—appeared to be associated with prosocial behaviours that were likely to be other-oriented—that did not simply reflect compliance with a request and had a cost. High levels of compliant prosocial behaviours in children of that age tend to be linked to non-assertiveness and proneness to personal distress (Eisenberg et al 1981, Eisenberg & Hand 1979, see Eisenberg & Fabes 1998).

In addition, spontaneous sharing, as assessed naturalistically in this study, has predicted prosocial behaviour and values/beliefs across childhood and into early adulthood. In follow-ups of the sample, prosocial constructs were assessed every two years from the ages of 9–10 into the 20s. In late childhood and adolescence, some behavioural measures of helping or sharing were obtained. Mothers' reports of children's prosocial behaviours were obtained in adolescence whereas friends reported on sympathy and prosocial tendencies in adulthood. We have found that spontaneous sharing in preschool was at least marginally correlated with costly donating or helping in childhood and adolescence; self-reported helping, consideration for others, prosocial values, and sympathy throughout adolescence and into adulthood; mothers' reports of helpfulness in adolescence; self-reported perspective taking in late adolescence and early adulthood; and friends' reports of sympathy or prosocial tendencies in early adulthood. Spontaneous sharing generally was unrelated to self-reported empathy in childhood, self-reported personal distress, low cost helping, and adult friends' reports of the study participants' perspective taking or specific, concrete prosocial behaviours (e.g. donated goods or clothes to a charity). In brief, spontaneous sharing in preschool was fairly consistently related to self-reports of prosocial responding and sympathy in late childhood, adolescence, and early adulthood, and sometimes predicted actual prosocial behaviour and mothers' reports thereof. There were few relations between the other types of prosocial behaviour and later prosocial responding, although preschoolers who were high in compliant sharing sometimes reported being relatively high in prosocial in adolescence and in the mid-20s. Of particular interest, reported sympathy generally tended to mediate the relations of preschoolers' spontaneous sharing to their prosocial tendencies in adulthood (Eisenberg et al 1999, 2002).

In addition, measures of self-reported prosociality, sympathy, and perspective taking were nearly always substantially related to the same or similar measures from up to 16 years earlier. These relations changed relatively little when controlling for social desirability. In addition, self-reported prosocial dispositions at adulthood generally were related to mothers' reports of children's prosocial behaviour in adolescence.

Empathy-related responding and moral reasoning

The roles of cognition and affect in morality—including moral reasoning—have been debated for many years. Cognitive developmental theorists have claimed that cognition and rationality are central to morality, and that the capabilities for complex perspective taking (cognitively taking the perspective of another) and for understanding abstract concepts are associated with, and underlie, advances in moral reasoning and in quality of prosocial behaviour (Colby et al 1983). Others have asserted that affect, especially empathy-related responding, often functions as a motive for other-oriented moral behaviour and can influence individuals' moral reasoning (Eisenberg 1986). We have argued moral reasoning reflects the beliefs and motives that guide moral decisions, including other-oriented concerns (Eisenberg 1986). Moreover, Hoffman (1987) has argued that sympathy/empathy stimulates the development of internalized moral reasoning reflecting concern for others' welfare, whereas I have proposed that sympathy primes the use of preexisting other-oriented moral cognitions (Eisenberg 1986). Based on such theoretical assertions, one would expect a relation between empathy-related responding, especially sympathy, and prosocial moral reasoning, and that prosocial moral reasoning sometimes might mediate the relation of sympathy to prosocial behaviour.

There is support for the association between sympathy and prosocial or care-oriented moral reasoning. For example, Skoe et al (2002) found an association between adults' reports of experiencing sympathy when resolving moral conflicts and their care-related moral reasoning, especially when discussing real-life dilemmas. In addition, reports of feelings of sympathy were related to ratings of the importance of a moral dilemma.

In addition, in our longitudinal study, we have repeatedly found relations between reported sympathy and higher level prosocial moral reasoning and/or the greater use of empathy-related types of moral reasoning and/or lesser use of hedonistic reasoning, from early adolescence into adulthood (e.g. Eisenberg et al 1991b, 1995). Furthermore, in a recent study of adolescents in Brazil, Eisenberg et al (2001a) obtained some initial support for the idea that prosocial moral reasoning mediates the relation of sympathy to prosocial behaviour. They found that sympathy (as well as cognitive perspective taking) predicted level of adolescents' prosocial moral reasoning, which in turn predicted their prosocial behaviour. Sympathy also had a direct path to prosocial behaviour. Thus, sympathy may contribute to prosocial behaviour directly, as well as through its effects on prosocial moral reasoning. In contrast, there was no evidence of a direct path from perspective taking to prosocial behaviour.

Empathy-related responding and antisocial behaviour and social competence

Theorists and researchers have argued that empathy/sympathy contributes not only to prosocial behaviour, but also to individual differences in antisocial behaviour and social competence. For example, people who tend to experience empathy when they perceive cues of others' negative emotion would be expected to inhibit behaviours that have hurtful effects for others. This argument is consistent with the recognition that deficits in empathy and remorse are common in individuals with antisocial personality disorders. Moreover, because empathy and sympathy would be expected to foster sensitivity to others and has been linked to greater prosocial behaviour, these vicarious reactions would be expected to contribute to children's social competence.

There is mounting support for the role of empathy and/or sympathy in antisocial behaviour and social competence (see Eisenberg et al 2006, Miller & Eisenberg 1988). For example, in a longitudinal study, Eisenberg et al (1996) found that teachers' reports of 6–8 year olds' dispositional sympathy were significantly correlated, concurrently and/or two years prior, with teacher-rated social skills and nonaggressive/socially appropriate behaviour, mothers' ratings of low levels of externalizing problems (including aggression and antisocial behaviour), and children's enacted and verbal socially competent responses in a puppet game in which they indicated what they would do in hypothetical social conflicts with peers. Four years later when the children were 10–12 years old, similar relations were found between teachers' reports of students' dispositional sympathy and measures of social competence concurrently and two, four and six years earlier, as well as with same-sex peers' reports of social status. Similarly, mothers' reports of children's dispositional sympathy were negatively related to mothers' and/or fathers' reports of externalizing problems (e.g. aggression, stealing) two, four and six years before, especially for boys (Murphy et al 1999). In a study of third graders in Indonesia, teachers' or parents' reports of children's dispositional sympathy tended to be associated with adults' and/or peers' reports of children's adjustment (i.e. low levels of externalizing problems) and popularity (Eisenberg et al 2001b). In a three-year follow-up, teacher-reported sympathy was still related to peer-reported liking, prosocial tendencies and low aggression, as well as teacher-reported social skills and adjustment, albeit primarily for boys.

Children's aggressive tendencies also have been correlated with situational measures of empathy-related responding. Zhou et al (2002) assessed elementary school children's facial and self-reported reactions to viewing mildly evocative slides of other people in positive or negative situations at two times, two years apart. In addition, parents' and teachers reported on the children's externalizing problem behaviours and social skills (i.e. socially appropriate behaviour and peer social status). At the first assessment, children's facial empathy (negative facial affect) in response to the slides depicting negative (but not positive) situations or others' facial expressions was negatively related to parents' and teachers' reports of children's externalizing problem behaviours; children's self-reported reactions were not related to their externalizing problems or social skills. Two years later, children's facial empathy to the negative slides and their self-reported empathy to both positive and negative slides (i.e., matching of the emotion in the slides) were associated with higher levels of adult-reported social skills and lower levels of adult-reported externalizing problems. In a structural equation model at the second assessment, empathy with the negative slides had stronger unique relations with children's social skills and low levels of externalizing problems than did empathy with positive slides, and this relation with problem behaviours held even when controlling for levels of empathy, social skills, and problem behaviours two years before.

Consistent with Zhou et al's (2002) findings, low levels of empathy may be especially important in the development of psychopathic tendencies and externalizing problems. Psychopaths or people with psychopathic traits appear to be less physiologically responsive to emotion-inducing stimuli (often mildly evocative slides) and to cues of others' distress than are non-psychopaths (Blair 1999). Thus, children who are not reactive to mild empathy-inducing stimuli may be at risk for externalizing problems. In a recent study, we (e.g. Liew et al 2003) found that boys (but not girls) who exhibited more heart rate or skin conductance responsivity when viewing slides depicting mild negative events or facial expressions were better regulated and had fewer externalizing problem behaviours than their less responsive peers. Because the stimuli were so mild, physiological arousal in this sample would not be expected to indicate personal distress (as it would in studies involving more evocative stimuli). It is important to keep in mind that either a lack of empathy or empathic overarousal (i.e. personal distress) may contribute to problems in moral and socioemotional development.

Summary

In summary, empathy, and especially sympathy, appear to play a major role in the development of other-oriented values, moral reasoning, and behaviour. There is considerable evidence that individual differences in the regulation of emotion are linked to individual differences in sympathetic and personally distressed reactions, and that both genetics and environment affect both regulation and empathy-related reactions (see Eisenberg et al 2006). Thus, interventions in families and schools are desirable to promote the development of sympathy and prosocial tendencies.

Acknowledgements

Much of the content of this chapter was adapted from Eisenberg (2005).

References

Batson CD 1991 The altruism question: Toward a social-psychological answer. Erlbaum, Hillsdale, NJ
Blair RJR 1999 Responsiveness to distress cues in the child with psychopathic tendencies. Pers Indiv Differ 27:135–145

Colby A, Kohlberg L, Gibbs J, Lieberman M 1983 A longitudinal study of moral judgment. Monographs of the Society for Research in Child Development, Serial No. 200, Vol. 48

Eisenberg N 1986 Altruistic emotion, cognition and behavior. Erlbaum, Hillsdale, NJ

Eisenberg N 2005 The development of empathy-related responding. In: Carlo G, Edwards CS (eds) Moral development through the lifespan: Theory, research and application. The 51st Nebraska on motivation. University of Nebraska Press, Lincoln, NE p73–117

Eisenberg N, Hand M 1979 The relationship of preschooler's reasoning about prosocial moral conflicts to prosocial behavior. Child Dev 50:356–363

Eisenberg N, Miller P 1987 The relation of empathy to prosocial and related behaviors. Psychol Bull 101:91–119

Eisenberg N, Fabes RA 1990 Empathy: conceptualization, assessment, and relation to prosocial behavior. Motiv Emotion 14:131–149

Eisenberg N, Fabes R 1998 Prosocial development. In: Damon W, Eisenberg N (eds) Handbook of child psychology, Vol 3, Social, emotional, and personality development (5th ed). Wiley, New York, p 701–778

Eisenberg N, Cameron E, Tryon K, Dodez R 1981 Socialization of prosocial behavior in the preschool classroom. Dev Psychol 17:773–782

Eisenberg N, Fabes RA, Schaller M, Carlo G, Miller PA 1991a The relations of parental characteristics and practices to children's vicarious emotional responding. Child Dev 62:1393–1408

Eisenberg N, Miller PA, Shell R, McNalley S, Shea C 1991b Prosocial development in adolescence: A longitudinal study. Dev Psychol 27:849–857

Eisenberg N, Carlo G, Murphy B, Van Court P 1995 Prosocial development in late adolescence: A longitudinal study. Child Dev 66:1179–1197

Eisenberg N, Fabes RA, Murphy BC, Karbon M, Smith M, Maszk P 1996 The relations of children's dispositional empathy-related responding to their emotionality, regulation, and social functioning. Dev Psychol 32:195–209

Eisenberg N, Guthrie IK, Murphy BC, Shepard SA, Cumberland A, Carlo G 1999 Consistency and development of prosocial dispositions: A longitudinal study. Child Dev 70: 1360–1372

Eisenberg N, Zhou Q, Koller S 2001a Brazilian adolescents' prosocial moral judgment and behavior: Relations to sympathy, perspective taking, gender-role orientation, and demographic characteristics. Child Dev 72:518–534

Eisenberg N, Liew J, Pidada S 2001b The relations of parental emotional expressivity with the quality of Indonesian children's social functioning. Emotion 1:107–115

Eisenberg N, Guthrie I, Cumberland A et al 2002 Prosocial development in early adulthood: A longitudinal study. J Pers Soc Psychol 82:993–1006

Eisenberg N, Fabes RA, Spinrad TL 2006 Prosocial behavior. In: Eisenbery N, Damon W, Lerner RM (eds), Handbook of child psychology, vol. 3: Social, emotional, and personality development (6th edn). Wiley, New York

Hoffman ML 1987 The contribution of empathy to justice and moral judgment. In N. Eisenberg & J. Strayer (eds), Empathy and its development. University of Cambridge Press, Cambridge p 47–80

Hoffman ML 2000 Empathy and moral development: Implications for caring and justice. Cambridge University Press, New York

Liew J, Eisenberg N, Losoya SH, Fabes RA, Guthrie IK, Murphy BC 2003 Children's physiological indices of empathy and their socioemotional adjustment: does caregivers' expressivity matter? J Fam Psychol 17:584–597

Miller P, Eisenberg N 1988 The relation of empathy to aggression and externalizing/antisocial behavior. Psychol Bull 103:324–344

Murphy BC, Shepard SA, Eisenberg N, Fabes RA, Guthrie IK 1999 Contemporaneous and
    longitudinal relations of dispositional sympathy to emotionality, regulation, and social func-
    tioning. J Early Adolescence 19:66–97
Skoe E, Eisenberg N, Cumberland A 2002 The role of reported emotion in real-life and hypo-
    thetical moral dilemmas. Pers Soc Psychol B 28:962–973
Underwood B, Moore B 1982 Perspective-taking and altruism. Psychol Bull 91:143–173
Zhou Q, Eisenberg N, Losoya SH et al 2002 The relations of parental warmth and positive
    expressiveness to children's empathy-related responding and social functioning: A longitu-
    dinal study. Child Dev 73:893–915

DISCUSSION

Silk: The stability of these children's responses is quite striking. One explanation
for this could be that children are early on rewarded for this positive behaviour in
a consistent fashion. Parents begin to treat them in a certain way and this becomes
part of who they are. The stability is generated by the environment in which they
are rewarded. What do the data tell us about the sources contributing to this
stability?

Spinrad: I don't want to speak directly to the stability, because I don't know
whether there is a relationship between socialization strategies and stability, *per se*.
However, there is evidence of a positive link between parental warmth and prosocial behaviour, sympathy and empathy (Deater-Deckard et al 2001, Kiang et al
2004, Kochanska et al 1999, Laible & Carlo 2004, Strayer & Roberts 2004), as well
as emotion regulation. Attachment security also has been found to relate to prosocial behaviour or sympathy (Waters et al 1986, Van der Mark et al 2002). Punitive
parenting tends to be negatively related to these behaviours (Asbury et al 2003,
Deater-Deckard et al 2001). We know that the parenting behaviours are likely to
be stable over time, and this could be contributing to the stability.

Warneken: You said the longitudinal study starts with four to five year olds. Are
there any longitudinal studies starting with children at a younger age? Hildy Ross
claimed that prosocial behaviours might decrease from young into middle childhood, but that was based upon cross-sectional data.

Spinrad: Nancy Eisenberg and Richard Fabes conducted a meta-analysis on age
changes and children's prosocial behaviours (Eisenberg & Fabes 1998). They
found prosocial behaviour increases with age in general, but these vary by the
context of the studies and with the age range. There are fewer studies in infancy
and toddlerhood; however, Zahn-Waxler and her colleagues have some evidence
that prosocial behaviour does increase in toddlerhood (Zahn-Waxler & Radke-
Yarrow 1982, Zahn-Waxler et al 1992, 2001), as do some others (Van der Mark et
al 2002, Lamb & Zekhireh 1997). In general, we see increases in prosocial behaviour with age, but the strength of these findings varies depending on the context
and the methods used (Eisenberg & Fabes 1998).

Hauser: You find correlations between the sympathy/empathy measures and the prosocial behaviour. Could something else be driving this correlation? One variable could be Walter Mischel's delayed gratification or discounting as a parameter, which does show up much earlier in development. He has studied these children from the age of about two, and this is a remarkably stable characteristic. Could this be the variable driving the correlation you are finding, rather than it being anything to do with sympathy or empathy?

Spinrad: Yes, we are very interested in the role of emotion regulation in children's prosocial behaviour and empathy/sympathy. We have also recently distinguished between regulation that is effortful versus less voluntary (Eisenberg & Spinrad 2004). In terms of the delay task, we might expect that the ability to delay would at least partly tap effortful regulation, although it might partly tap children's low impulsivity as well (Spinrad et al 2006). Regardless of that issue, there have been quite a few data that tell us that children who are relatively well-regulated are more likely to behave prosocially (Eisenberg et al 1996, 1997) and to experience sympathy as opposed to personal distress reactions (Eisenberg & Fabes 1995, Eisenberg et al 1996, Eisenberg et al 2001). We believe that this behaviour is probably underlying some of the ability to be other-oriented as opposed to being self-focused.

Hauser: The nice thing about the species of monkey we work on is that they twin naturally, making DZ twins. We have begun to look at heritability of these kinds of behaviour, to see if there is consistency across different tasks. Animals that are patient in one task may well be patient in others. When you do Walter Michel's delayed gratification tasks, are the children who hold on longer the ones who are more prosocial? It could be the impulsivity level that is driving the prosocial behaviour and sympathy/empathy is just an intermediate variable, correlated because of the delayed gratification.

Spinrad: I would argue that sympathy is mediating a relation between emotional regulation and prosocial behaviours.

Sigman: Didn't the data you presented earlier about heritability speak to that?

Spinrad: There is an interesting study by Robinson et al (2001). Using a twin-design sample, the researchers examined toddlers' responses to feigned distress in several situations, when the victim was either a stranger or the mother. Their findings showed that the heritability of prosocial behaviour depended on whether the victim was the mother or the stranger (with a stronger heritability index toward the stranger).

Frank: Some evidence suggests that criminals were overwhelmingly likely to have had impulse control problems as children. It could be that there is some independent competence called the ability to delay gratification, but causation could go in the other direction, too. If you think about the repeated prisoner's dilemma, a purely prudent person would want to cooperate on the first round to maintain a string of successful interactions. The difficulty is that the gain comes now if you defect, whereas the reward for cooperating comes only in the future. If you had some independent concern for the well-being of your trading partner, it would be easier to clear the impulse-control hurdle

Hauser: I find the discounting issue interesting, and am convinced by our tamarin results. The problem is not the understanding of the pay-offs of cooperation, but rather the inability to delay gratification. It could very well be that all animals are capable of perceiving the advantages of reciprocity, but simply fail to engage in such cooperative behaviour because they are incapable of waiting for returned rewards. Impatience causes reciprocity to crash.

Warneken: At the beginning you distinguished prosocial from altruistic behaviours, yet when you presented the data altruistic behaviours didn't show up any more. Is that because altruistic behaviour was so infrequent it was collapsed with prosocial behaviours in a broader sense?

Spinrad: The differentiation between prosocial and altruistic behaviours is in regard to motivation. Because it is difficult to assess children's motivation, we refer to all of the behaviours we measure as prosocial behaviours.

Warneken: But in the definitions it seems like a continuous variable on one dimension, with prosocial on one side and altruism on the other. There is no cut-off point where you would say now it is totally altruistic behaviour.

Spinrad: Again, I would argue that the difference is the motivation behind the behaviour, which is difficult to assess. Some behaviours are altruistic whereas some are not, but we simply have difficulty differentiating among them because we do not know the child's thoughts, goals and motives.

Warneken: Alright, according to what you just said, prosocial behaviour can be assessed by looking at the behaviour alone without looking at the motives. When you then want to find out whether it is altruistic or not you have to look at the motives. But it rather seemed to me that it is all about motives here, and only if the motives are identified and they are all about the other can we say it is altruistic.

Spinrad: Yes. Prosocial behaviour is a more general term, referring to behaviours such as volunteering, helping, sharing and comforting. Altruism is a specific case of this type of prosocial behaviour that is other-oriented (Eisenberg 1986).

Blair: I want to return to the delay of gratification and impulse control questions. The disadvantage of having this as the link between empathy and prosocial behaviour is that one of the measures was the emotional response to the pictures. This index of the basic emotional response is unlikely to relate to delay of gratification in the way that it is usually thought about. It would be difficult to link these two. Regarding the impulse control, we can be pretty sure that impulse control more generally is not the thing that is driving empathy because you have children with attention deficit hyperactivity disorder (ADHD), a classic impulse control disorder, and they are not showing indications of profound empathy impairment. We can be confident that this is not the explanation.

Van Lange: Research on the prisoner's dilemma confirms that the orientation with the future is quite independent of prosocial orientation. Some people with an individualistic orientation can take long-term orientation and be cooperative. One reason why pure reciprocity elicits a lot of cooperation is that people cooperate because they know in the long run it is a good thing to do, but these are not people who are inherently prosocial.

Gallese: Is there any relationship between sympathy, the development of prosocial behaviour and the specific type of attachment these children experience?

Spinrad: There is some work that suggests that children who are securely attached are more likely to be empathic, but much of work doesn't differentiate between empathy and sympathy (Van der Mark et al 2002). On a related issue, I have some data showing that maternal sensitivity/responsivity observed at 10 months of age predicts sympathy toward their mother and a stranger at 18 months of age (Spinrad & Stifter 2006). This study doesn't directly assess security of attachment, but given the existing links between maternal responsivity and attachment security, these findings are related to your question.

Montague: When you do an experiment like that, how do you tell which way it is going? I may be being more sensitive to my baby because it is eliciting this behaviour from me. The baby may be selecting for parental behaviour rather than the mother sending signals to the baby that induce a different state in the baby.

Spinrad: It is easier to be sensitive to some babies than others, I agree. So, it is important to take the child's characteristics into account. However, I think that sensitivity is a code that takes the child's behaviour into account. For example, if the child is focusing on a particular toy, a sensitive mother would also focus on that toy and not move onto another toy until the child lost attention to that toy. Moreover, if a child is fussy, a mother can be sensitive by soothing and comforting that child.

Montague: A child's behaviour is difficult to characterize. It indexes a certain part of the parental behavioural space. This is why children with autism spectrum disorders are particularly hard on parents, because the parents are expecting a whole range of responses from the child which they don't get.

Spinrad: I don't think that there is any question that there are bidirectional effects. In fact, a study by Eisenberg and colleagues found that parental behaviour predicted children's emotion regulation over time (controlling for early emotion regulation). In turn, children's emotion regulation predicted parenting behaviours two years later (even after controlling for early levels of the behaviour). Thus, it is clear that parents influence their children as well as the reverse (i.e. children influence their parents).

Gergely: With respect to the question about attachment security, the data that are contradicting the idea that the quality of attachment would be solely infant- or temperament-induced (see Vaughn & Bost 1999) are the findings that indicate no (or only very low) correlation between the types of attachment (secure, avoidant, resistant or disorganized) that characterize an infant's relationship to different caregivers, respectively. A child can be securely attached to one attachment figure while showing insecure attachment in relation to the other. Also, the type of the parent's attachment status as measured by the Adult Attachment Interview (AAI) (George et al 1996) predicts rather well the infant's specific attachment classification with the parent at one year of age (as measured by the Ainsworth Strange Situation Test, see Ainsworth et al 1978) (Fonagy et al 1991). Temperament (child → parent effects) seems an inadequate account of this finding as the AAI of the parent is collected and coded before the birth of the child.

Singer: I'm trying to take a neuroscientific perspective on your research on empathy and fit your data into this account. The easy neuroscientific story would be to suggest that the better your action perception resonance mechanism in your brain, the more you share the feelings of others and the more empathic you are. This would imply, however, that sharing negative emotions with others lead automatically to own distress. Now you are showing negative correlations between personal distress and helping behaviour, the latter again associated with empathy. According to such a view, any resonance mechanism resulting in personal distress by the sight of someone suffering negative emotions is hindering empathy.

Now you are also saying that psychopaths don't respond as sensitively to emotional stimuli as normal controls, and this is why they aren't empathic. This seems to suggest in turn, that sharing affect with the others is a necessary condition for empathy to arise. In conclusion, I would suggest that you need both for empathy to arise: first a shared representation mechanism to allow for sharing affective experiences with others and, in addition, a top–down modulation mechanism which allows to suppress to strong empathic responses so that you can engage in helping behaviour.

Spinrad: I think there is an optimal level of distress. Eisenberg et al (1994) proposed that emotional overarousal would be associated with personal distress whereas moderate distress is associated with sympathy. Hoffman (1982) also has made this suggestion. Thus, if people can maintain arousal in a tolerable range, they should experience sympathy. There is empirical work to support this notion (Eisenberg et al 1991). Also, distress can be related to helping, when it is the easiest way to reduce one's own distress (for example, when a person cannot escape the distressed other).

Singer: Here neuroscience can make a distinction between pure cognitive perspective taking and empathizing. The first is based on different brain structures than the latter. It seemed that you were saying that sympathy is just engaging the perspective taking network or theory of mind network, which is totally different from the empathy system which is based on limbic brain structures rather than pre-frontal structures or temporoparietal junction (TPJ). But I didn't get the impression that you were really suggesting that. You said that one part of sympathy is actually based on an empathic response (that is, feeling the same thing as the other person does). That would clearly involve brain structures associated with the processing of bodily or sensory experiences rather than merely structures dealing with propositional attitudes.

Spinrad: It is feeling concern or sorrow for the other person. It may stem from feeling what the other person feels.

C Frith: Can't you say that it is all a matter of degree? There is social distress if your response is too great. At the beginning of the meeting I suggested that if you see someone sad and you feel sad, this initiates in you the need to take action to reduce your sadness. In the same way, this could lead you to act to reduce the other person's sadness, which will reduce your sadness because of the resonance.

Singer: I would say that sympathy arises because you have the ability for top–down control of your feelings. All the difference observed between sympathetic or non-sympathetic children should then be in whether these children have affective emotional regulation mechanisms in place.

Moll: It depends on the measure that you use. What was your measure of 'sympathy'?

Spinrad: We used three different measures: self report, facial measures and physiological measures. Facial concern is related to prosocial behaviour, but there is a level of distress that we consider an over-arousal, where children will be more focused on their own arousal and alleviating their own distress than being able to act on this and behave prosocially. In such studies, children can easily escape dealing with the other person who induced the empathy, so there is no need to help to reduce their own arousal.

Sigman: I have a question about gender differences. This area of research seems marked by very large gender differences. First, there is a big primary effect of femininity on the whole process, and then there are differences in stability over time, where it sounds like you are getting more prediction from males than females. How do you understand and interpret these gender differences.

Spinrad: Again, Eisenberg & Fabes (1998) conducted a meta-analysis on gender differences as well. Findings showed that gender differences seem to be stronger depending on the type of measure used. Self-report measures produce much stronger sex differences, whereas facial or physiological measures of empathy, sympathy or personal distress show weaker sex differences.

Sigman: What about stability? Does this continue to be stronger for males?

Spinrad: I don't know.

Blair: I have a comment about the personal distress/empathy differentiation. The potential differentiation isn't to do with the level of arousal to get to the negative affect, but the fact that one set of children have a set of strategies to deal with the problem facing them while another set don't. There's a good example of this, which I haven't seen published, where researchers took young children and put them in an empathy-inducing paradigm in which the researcher feigns hurting themselves. They taught one set of children to mop the experimenter with a cloth but not the other set. The non-taught children showed significantly higher levels of crying and confusion. The sad face is an aversive stimulus. The difference is, if you can deal with it and take away the sad face you are in a relief condition as opposed to a situation where you have no idea what to do. There is a way of characterizing the personal distress/empathy divide that is more compatible with the sorts of things you were going for.

Silk: I have a question about the distribution of these traits in children. Is this a bimodal distribution? How does this follow along these dimensions that you mentioned?

Spinrad: Children can experience both sympathy and personal distress. We show them sympathy-inducing films and some children will experience sympathy, and others experience more personal distress, but they can experience both, likely sequentially. We don't look at this as a distribution.

Silk: When you have your correlations, you must be putting something in for the different time periods for each child.

Spinrad: We look at the film, decide what the sympathy-inducing portion is, and decide what the distress-inducing portion is. We look to see whether children experience distress during the sympathy portion.

Silk: What does that distribution look like?

Spinrad: I don't know, but distress responses generally are more common than concern reactions, in the baseline and during the evocative portions of the film.

Frank: Some evidence suggests that criminals were overwhelmingly likely to have had impulse control problems as children. It could be that there is some independent competence called the ability to delay gratification, but causation could go in the other direction, too. If you think about the repeated prisoner's dilemma, a purely prudent person would want to cooperate on the first round to maintain a string of successful interactions. The difficulty is that the gain comes now if you defect, whereas the reward for cooperating comes only in the future. If you had some independent concern for the well-being of your trading partner, it would be easier to clear the impulse-control hurdle?

Spinrad: I think it has to do with the amount of cost. If we did control it, I think we'd find the same with both. In some of Nancy Eisenberg's work with children, helping was operationalized as low cost behaviours whereas sharing involved giving up territory or a possession.

References

Ainsworth MDS, Blehar MC, Waters E, Wall S 1978 Patterns of attachment: a psychological study of the strange situation. Lawrence Erlbaum, Hillsdale, NJ

Asbury K, Dunn JF, Pike A, Plomin R 2003 Nonshared environmental influences on individual differences in early behavioral development: A monozygotic twin differences study. Child Dev 74:933–943

Deater-Deckard K, Dunn J, O'Connor TG, Davies L, Golding J and the ALSPAC Study Team 2001 Using the stepfamily genetic design to examine gene-environmental processes in child and family functioning. Marriage Family Rev 33:131–156

Eisenberg N 1986 Altruistic emotion, cognition, and behavior. Hillsdale, N.J: Erlbaum.

Eisenberg N, Fabes RA 1995 The relation of young children's vicarious emotional responding to social competence, regulation, and emotionality. Cognit Emotion 9:203–228

Eisenberg N, Fabes R 1998 Prosocial development. In: Damon W, Eisenberg N (eds) Handbook of child psychology, Vol 3, Social, emotional, and personality development (5th ed). Wiley, New York, p 701–778

Eisenberg N, Spinrad TL 2004 Emotion-related regulation: Sharpening the definition. Child Dev 75:334–339

Eisenberg N, Fabes RA, Murphy B et al 1994 The relations of emotionality and regulation to dispositional and situational empathy-related responding. J Personal Social Psychol 66:776–797

Eisenberg N, Fabes RA, Karbon M et al 1996 The relations of children's dispositional prosocial behavior to emotionality, regulation, and social functioning. Child Dev 67:974–992

Eisenberg N, Fabes RA, Schaller M et al 1991 Personality and socialization correlates of vicarious emotional responding. J Personal Social Psychol 61:459–470

Eisenberg N, Guthrie IK, Fabes RA et al 1997 The relations of regulation and emotionality to resiliency and competent social functioning in elementary school children. Child Dev 68:295–311

Fonagy P, Steele H, Steele M 1991 Maternal representations of attachment during pregnancy predict the organization of infant-mother attachment at one year of age. Child Dev 62:891–905

George C, Kaplan N, Main M 1996 The adult attachment interview protocol, 3rd edn, Department of Psychology, University of California at Berkeley, Unpublished manuscript

Hoffman ML 1982 Development of prosocial motivation: Empathy and guilt. In: Eisenberg N (ed) The development of prosocial behavior. Academic Press, New York, p 281–313

Kiang L, Moreno AJ, Robinson JL 2004 Maternal preconceptions about parenting predict child temperament, maternal sensitivity, and children's empathy. Devel Psychol 6:1081–1092

Kochanska G, Forman DR, Coy KC 1999 Implications of the mother–child relationship in infancy for socialization in the second year of life. Infant Behav Dev 22:249–265

Lamb S, Zakhireh B 1997 Toddlers' attention to the distress of peers in a day care setting. Early Edu Dev 8:105–118

Robinson JL, Zahn-Waxler C, Emde RN 2001 Relationship context as a moderator of sources of individual difference in empathic development. In: Emde RN, Hewitt JK (eds) Infancy to early childhood: genetic and environmental influences on developmental change. Oxford University Press, p 257–268

Spinrad TL, Stifter CA 2006 Empathy-related responding to distress in toddlers: predictions from negative emotionality and maternal behaviour in infancy. Infancy, in press

Spinrad TL, Eisenberg N, Gaertner BM 2006 Measures of effortful regulation in young children. Infant Mental Health J, in press

Strayer J, Roberts W 2004 Children's anger, emotional expressiveness, and empathy: Relations with parents' empathy, emotional expressiveness, and parenting practices. Social Dev 13:229–254

Van der Mark IL, van Ijzendoorn MH, Bakermans-Kranenburg MJ 2002 Development of empathy in girls during the second year of life: Associations with parenting, attachment, and temperament. Social Dev 11:451–468

Vaughn BE, Bost KK 1999 Attachment and temperament. In: Cassidy J, Shaver PR (eds) Handbook of attachment: theory, research, and clinical applications. Guilford, New York, p 198–225

Waters E, Hay D, Richters J 1986 Infant–parent attachment and the origins of prosocial and antisocial behavior. In: Olweus D, Block J, Radke-Yarrow M (eds) Development of antisocial and prosocial behavior: Research, theories, and issues. Academic Press, Orlando, p 97–125

Zahn-Waxler C, Radke-Yarrow M 1982 The development of altruism: Alternative research strategies. In: Eisenberg N (ed) The development of prosocial behaviour. Academic Press, New York, p 109–137

Zahn-Waxler C, Robinson J, Emde RN 1992 The development of empathy in twins. Dev Psychol 28:1038–1047

Zahn-Waxler C, Schiro K, Robinson JL, Emde RN, Schmitz S 2001 Empathy and prosocial patterns in young MZ and DZ Twins: Development and genetic and environmental influences. In: R. N. Emde, J. K. Hewitt (eds) Infancy to early childhood. Oxford University Press, p 141–162

GENERAL DISCUSSION I

C Frith: I suggested at the beginning that perhaps part of what this meeting is about is to think about what emotions are for. Marc Hauser, you seem to be suggesting that they are an epiphenomenon!

Hauser: I didn't say that they are not useful. The question is whether they are there to drive the moral decision, or whether the moral decision happens and then the emotions follow from that.

C Frith: What happens after the emotions? How are they useful?

Hauser: They drive behaviour. The question is whether the judgement of a permissible action drives or is being driven by an emotional state. The psychopath case is the clearest. My prediction is that psychopaths have complete moral competence, but when it comes to acting on a decision they will go wrong because there is no emotional check on the behaviour. The emotions are not motivating what we would consider to be morally appropriate behaviour.

Montague: How would you distinguish that from a psychopath who had an emotional reaction and then acted on it inappropriately?

Blair: They don't have these sorts of emotional reactions.

Hauser: The reason they get into trouble is not because they have weird views about what is right and wrong, but because when it comes to actually doing something or refraining from it, they lack the emotional checks and balances on behaviour that non-psychopaths have.

Blair: This is not an accurate description of the data. The moral/conventional distinction shows that they do have weird viewpoints about what is right and wrong. They show less of a differentiation between moral and conventional transgressions. Your model suggests that emotion comes after the judgement, but here we have a case of an emotion based disorder where moral judgement is disturbed. You have to give an alternative account as to why they show impairment on the moral/conventional distinction task. This is a task that healthy children pass from the age of four. Individuals with psychopathy don't have executive function/dorsolateral prefrontal cortex problems. You need a model as to what else could be driving the fact that they don't understand the moral/conventional distinction.

Hauser: The tests that we want to do are very different from what you have done. As I mentioned briefly before, none of your tasks in the moral-conventional distinction set up situations where either the action or the omission will lead to a harmful or helpful consequence, and where straightforward deontological or utilitarian principles work straight off. So they are different kinds of dilemmas and I believe that people have worked out the psychology of these in a more rigorous way than for the moral-conventional distinction which I find fuzzier.

Gergely: I think this relates to what Chris Frith was saying at the beginning. The language analogy breaks down when it comes to morality, in so far as why would evolution produce a set of automatic rules for judgement and not for behaviour?

Hauser: I think you are thinking about language in terms of communication. This is not how I am thinking about language: I am making the deeper analogy, which is that moral behaviour is to communication as moral competence is to the language faculty. The knowledge that we bring computationally to language may or may not be used for communication. I can do all sorts of things that are not communication with parts of that faculty, in the same way that I can imagine actions without doing them. Why is this a challenge for evolution?

Gergely: The difference is that in the case of language there is a strong argument from the impoverished input for the need for the system to acquire language. You have to postulate the same central function for your moral system: that it is there to enable the acquisition of the capacity for moral judgements. Language is used for communication, and moral judgements are used for guiding moral behaviour.

Hauser: I agree. Moral judgements are used for behaviour: sometimes they will match and sometimes they won't. It is true that the language faculty is used for communication, but it is used for other things too. In the same way, whatever the computation is that runs over the consequences of action and generates a judgement, it is used for lots of other things too. My guess is that the moral faculty is a hodge podge or kluge of different capacities of the mind. Intention and action is not privileged to morality, nor are emotions.

C Frith: I don't understand why you can't go straight from judgement to behaviour. What does the intermediate step of emotion add?

Hauser: I'm not sure it necessarily adds anything, and one of my goals is to challenge what I see as an untested assumption by many in the field, where emotions are considered to be the driving force, without considering alternative accounts of the sources of our moral judgments. Making the analogy to language opens these alternative possibilities up. We can think of strong and weak versions of this analogy. The first is purely heuristic, allowing us to raise and explore brand new questions. Then there is the stronger analogy where we ask about the possibility that the moral and language faculties work in precisely the same way, though with different functions and conceptual content. One issue that emerges when we consider the stronger analogy is the extent to which each of these computational faculties can be penetrated by other systems of the mind, especially our beliefs, and whether we have access to any of the principles that are operative in guiding our judgments. Here we just don't know, but there are hints that certain aspects of our moral judgments may work like our linguistic judgments: automatically and without access to the underlying principles. Someone raised the question of development.

Chomsky could ask the developmental question in language because linguists had already begun to characterize the key descriptive principles of language, the principles that can account for knowledge in the mature state. We don't have this level of descriptive adequacy with morality, so we can't pose the questions about development or address what is often called the level of explanatory adequacy. All we can ask is whether there is a sense that the input to the child is impoverished relative to what is coming out. We lack information on the description of the state in the adult. With regard to emotion, it is an issue of the temporal course of events. No one is denying that emotions play some role in morality. The question is where emotions play a role. James Blair would say that the conventional moral distinction may be one of the cases which I can't account for. I am sure there are a lot of things that I can't account for. But at this point, the literature is very unclear about whether emotions are the stuff of all of our intuitive moral judgments, or derivative, even epiphenomenal. Further, for all of the cases that I have presented here, we don't yet know whether the emotions are epiphenomenal, or involved in generating the judgment. But now that the distinctions are being clarified, we can begin to do the necessary work.

C Frith: The other point I'd like to make is to what extent are you just talking about decision making? When does the moral component come into decision making, or is morality simply decision making in a social context? Is this just a continuum, or is there something special about moral judgements?

Van Lange: What makes morality is the social aspect of decision making. Morality would have no meaning for Robinson Crusoe. Only after Friday came along social emotions became useful and meaningful. Where do emotions play a role? Before or after cognition? I can imagine examples where emotions start and then cognition follows. What are emotions for? I think they regulate collectives and groups. Guilt is often harmful for yourself, but for the collective it is a good thing.

Montague: How would you rank incest taboos? There is a kind of genetic calculus based that is behind this, which pollutes to an extent the explanation that you need social interactions for a moral judgement.

C Frith: Is an incest taboo moral or conventional?

Blair: It comes in as a subcategory of disgust-based moral transgressions.

Montague: That's how you implement them, but I'm talking about categorizing them.

Moll: It depends on cultural issues to a degree. It is a feature which is highly biologically based, but there are cultures which allow it.

Silk: No, it's a consistent taboo.

Brosnan: It's also consistent across many species.

Montague: We have biological expediency (propagating your DNA with enough fidelity into the next generation) and social alignment. Those vectors are pointing in the same direction. I'd throw away the moral norm piece and say that the biological expediency grew into a social norm.

Blair: The reason for having two is that there are individuals impaired with respect to care-based morality but not disgust-based morality

Gallese: What is your favoured ontogenetic developmental scenario for moral competence?

Hauser: One that would look like language. There is a set of innate, universal principles that constrain the range of observed variation, with each culture providing the relevant input to tune up or set all the relevant parameters.

Frank: Selected for the ability to do what that is beneficial to the organism?

Hauser: I am not even sure they were selected to do anything beneficial for the organism. They are going to operate over actions that are presumably cooperative and social in some sense, but they could be by-products of computations that evolved for some other reason.

Gallese: Are they totally genetically determined?

Hauser: Aspects of the computational parts will be genetically determined, and then local culture experiences will tune up through instruction the particular moral system.

Gallese: You said earlier you don't see any reason to envisage a moral faculty as such in the brain. So what would make this genetically determined computational procedure specific for moral competence? I agree there is no reason to believe that there must be a specific system for moral competence that has evolved in the brain. But if moral competence is not a socially learned process and is genetically determined, what makes this computational device so specific?

Hauser: Well, of course it has to be in the brain as opposed to in some other part of my body. I don't think morality is some arbitrary, completely cultural artefact. The study of morality, like the study of language, is part of biology, and part of this study will include analyses of the brain. In terms of competence, I think that you have to do is what James Blair started doing, asking questions about the difference between a social convention and a moral rule. There is a nice example by Shaun Nichols (Nichols 2002), addressing what it takes to change something from being merely a social convention to being a moral rule. His idea is that you take something that is a convention and marry it to a strong emotion like disgust. You are at a dinner party when your host announces that those people feeling sick should feel free to spit their phlegm into the wine glasses. When people are asked whether the host can dictate like this, most people say that he can not. They treat the case like a moral transgression as opposed to a social or conventional transgression. Authority can overrule conventions but not moral rules. Conventions bound with disgust turn into moral rules. To flesh out this claim, James Blair will be testing young psychopaths, and we are testing Huntington's chorea patients who selectively lack a disgust response.

Dupoux: It seems to me that there are two ways of looking at emotions. There is one type of emotion that is necessary for the judgement, which is the emotion that the person outside is experiencing. If I give you poison intentionally you will suffer a lot, and this will clearly affect moral judgement, as opposed to if I give you a cookie and you are OK. The emotion experienced by the victim will be the input of the judgement. It is different from the emotion that I as a judge am experiencing.

Hauser: I am not saying that you don't experience emotions that might not affect what you do. Your example doesn't address what I said. I'm arguing that if you tell me that person A got poison and person B got a cookie, I'll code that as someone getting something bad and someone getting something good. There's no emotion in the equation.

Dupoux: To compute what is good and what is bad you have to take into account that harm was done to someone. You have to be able to compute what is harm and what is not. To do this, the emotional state of the person who is experiencing harm or not experiencing harm must be taken into account.

Hauser: Why?

Dupoux: How else would you do it?

Hauser: By pure association.

Blair: The problem you are facing is why harm to another should be of interest to you. One way of doing this is to say that you have set your system up so that aversion to another's harm is a default value. The problem with that view is that this would be the only negatively valenced entity that I can think of that has nothing to do with emotion.

Dupoux: I'm thinking about a child. They need to know what is harm and what is not harm. The way they can know this is by interpreting emotions. If someone is crying, this is a cue suggesting that harm has been done to that person.

Hauser: Take the example of the lexicon. If I couldn't speak French, I wouldn't know what the word *chaise* means. Now follow the same logic: we can put in pieces that count as nouns or verbs, but ultimately the computation is going to run over that. The analogy to language is not that there can't be any input. There has to be input. The question is, once the child sees something that makes someone cry, has she coded a simple emotional association between the act and a negative consequence, or has she analysed, unconsciously of course, aspects of the event that lie beneath the surface, focused on the causal structure of actions and consequences, the mental states of the agents, including their beliefs and goals. If the latter is correct, then, again, judgments derive from the causal–intentional aspects of the event with emotions arising out of this analysis.

Blair: As soon as you are talking about negative and positive you are talking about emotion.

Hauser: Not at all. Actions could be parameterized as plus and minus, with no emotion. Just think of the pluses and minuses as DO or DON'T DO. Again, no emotion, even though we may bind emotions to these valenced actions, and these may help in memory and even in motivation of action.

Blair: We use facial expression information to communicate our socialization. This strongly pushes forwards an emotional point of view. This is the problem that the old rational viewpoints have. Why do we make these differences between particular types of rules? Why do we use all this affect when we are trying to socialize children?

Montague: What aren't these not just variables? Are we viewing them as some extra quality that I am not understanding?

Sigman: Isn't there something wrong with the reward system in psychopaths, in that psychopaths will do harm for pleasure?

Blair: That's not correct. There is no increased incidence of sadism among psychopaths relative to the rest of the criminal population.

Sigman: There has to be some sort built-in mechanism for why emotion is even important to a child.

Hauser: This is not a denial of the role of emotion. You can't have an emotion before the evaluative or appraisal system calculates some aspect of the event or action, even if it is a trivial as categorizing the object. How can you have an emotion unless you have an evaluative system give you the emotion?

Sigman: What if you don't pay attention to that, and don't perceive it?

Hauser: The question is, what is giving you the lack of response to emotion? Is it because you have no emotion or because you have a deficit in your mechanism for perceiving? Do they fail because they fail to appraise the situation that would generate the emotion? This would be the way I would think about it.

Gallese: Motivation is frequently determined by social referencing. It is not something that is inborn, but is something you learn to calibrate.

Hauser: One question is, are there mechanisms in place that take certain kinds of input as relevant or not?

Singer: If you could train someone to have a moral evaluation without ever having to respond to it, would you ever have an emotion attached to it. In imaging research, could we find out where the emotion centre is? We would predict that there are some moral evaluations that don't have an emotion as an epiphenomenon when they have never been attached to any action. You could falsify your theory by showing examples of fairness evaluation where you show emotion-related limbic systems even where people didn't have to make a judgement or act on it.

Hauser: Chris Frith asked me whether we could get our moral dilemmas to the level of real world cases. I think the economic games that have been put forward in this conference, and in the entire field of behavioural economics and neuroeconomics, are equally artificial. There are problems going both directions. Given the kinds of claims that have been made about emotional deficits, if it turns out that our patient populations are significantly damaged on these dilemmas then this part of my theory is in trouble. To me there are two issues. First, how does the appraisal mechanism work, period? Second, where does the emotion come into the story?

Singer: Would you predict emotion coming in if there is no action necessary?

Hauser: Is that a real possibility?

Frank: What about a hypothetical question about a moral dilemma?

Singer: Just imagine this Gedanken experiment. If you had to make a judgement and there would never have been an action associated with it, would you also get emotions as an epiphenomenon of such a judgement?

Hauser: No. This is where the hunter-gatherers will be of interest, because many of the dilemmas we use are situations where there is action at a distance. Hunter-gatherers have no concept of this. That is, when they act, it is with immediate consequences: helping someone sick who is here, in the tribe, or harming someone by physical contact, or at best, a spear or arrow, but the latter were relatively recent inventions. When hunter-gathers are confronted with dilemmas that require an assessment of an action with a consequence that is either physically or temporally at a distance, what kind of judgment will this trigger? If it triggers the same architecture, then I think we are in a far stronger position to argue that there are evolutionarily ancient, innate principles, that set up a range of possible outcomes, a range of possible moral systems.

Frank: One of the variants of the trolley experiment is to push the fat guy off the bridge onto the tracks below. People are reluctant to do this, even though they would flip the switch without hesitation. The difference in the proportion of people who reach the judgement that the fat man should be used to derail the trolley has to be explained as part of the emotional reaction to the idea of pushing a fat man off the bridge.

Hauser: I have an anecdote that provides one kind of answer to your question. My father was a very distinguished theoretical physicist. I told him about the kind of research I was doing, and I gave him the bystander case to begin with. He said you should flick the switch because it is five versus one. Then I gave him the fat man case and he said of course you push the fat man. I found this interesting, because few people give this answer. Then I said that you are a doctor in a hospital and an ambulance has come in with five people who are badly hurt. Each needs an organ, and there's no time to send out for organ donation, but a healthy person has walked in and you could take his organs. He says that this isn't OK, even though it is sacrificing one person to save five. I point out that he just pushed the fat guy off the bridge. He then changed his mind about the fat case, and pretty soon, the bystander case unravels as well, leaving my poor father without a rational way of working out a solution. Now one could say that the organ case involves a little more emotion than the fat man case and this is why about 10% of our population will kill the fat guy, but only about 1% will kill the innocent hospital visitor. The question is: can an emotional difference explain all of this, any of this?

Frank: What would you say?

Hauser: I would say that both cases can be explained by the doctrine of the double effect, with the emotions following. Again, and to reiterate my broken record mantra, I want to try and push as hard as I can the idea that there is an appraisal system—a universal moral grammar—that evaluates each event in terms of a cold calculus, operating over the causal and intentional structure of the event. This system may or may not then trigger an emotion, and this emotion may or may not arise before or after the judgment. Bring on the evidence.

Reference

Nichols S 2002 Norms with feeling: toward a psychological account of moral judgment. Cognition 84:221–236

A social interaction analysis of empathy and fairness

Paul A. M. Van Lange*, Marcello Gallucci†, Johan C. Karremans‡, Anthon Klapwijk* and Chris Reinders Folmer*

*Department of Social Psychology, Free University, Amsterdam, The Netherlands, †University of Milan, Italy, ‡Radboud University, Nijmegen, The Netherlands

Abstract. This paper advances a social interaction analysis of altruism, as a likely result of empathy, and egalitarianism, as a key component of fairness. A social interaction analysis is unique in that it (a) focuses on the persons and the situation, (b) includes proximal and distal influences (such as personality and relational influences, as well as cognitive and emotional processes), (c) yields action-reaction patterns that are largely observable and therefore especially relevant to learning, and (d) helps conceptualize interpersonal orientations that affect behaviour and social interactions. The chapter discusses the ubiquity of altruism and egalitarianism in the context of social dilemmas and related situations, and concludes that these two orientations are important to theorizing and research in various disciplines that seek to understand the motivational underpinnings of social interactions in dyads and groups.

2006 Empathy and Fairness. Wiley, Chichester (Novartis Foundation Symposium 278) p 97–110

A social interaction analysis of empathy and fairness

Are people good and bad? Are people basically selfish, or would it be more accurate to characterize human nature by a broader set of interpersonal orientations? The dominating view in science on human nature has been that people primarily or exclusively pursue self-interest, with little or no regard for the well-being of others. Indeed, philosophers, such as Thomas Hobbes, or economists such as Adam Smith, may easily come to mind, even though the assumption of rational self-interest is widespread among various scientific fields and disciplines. Even within psychology, there are longstanding concepts such as the 'pursuit of pleasure' in psychoanalytic theory, 'utility' in models of social decision-making, or 'reinforcement' in theories of learning and behaviour modification, which are rooted in the assumption of self-interest. And most people tend to rely on a belief in 'selfishness' when making judgments or when seeking to understand social behaviour.

We suggest that the assumption of rational self-interest is too limited to account for interpersonal behaviour. In fact, like Miller (1999), we think that it is a biased

97

scheme that many people use as a framework for interpreting others' behaviour, but not their own behaviour or that of others close to them. Indeed, there is good deal of evidence indicating that people think of themselves as better than others, especially on attributes that are strongly linked to selfishness, such as being 'good', being honest, and the like (e.g. Van Lange & Sedikides 1998). A more accurate representation of human nature can be derived from theorizing and research on interpersonal orientations (Kelley & Thibaut 1978, Van Lange 1999). In recent conceptualizations, a typology of six interpersonal orientations is advanced, designed to help us understand the basic decision rules (or motives) that people adopt in their interpersonal dealings. These orientations include: (a) altruism, enhancement of other's outcomes, (b) cooperation, enhancement of own and other's outcomes (or joint outcomes), (c) equality, minimization of absolute differences between own and other's outcomes, (d) individualism, enhancement of own outcomes, (e) competition, enhancement of relative advantage over other's outcomes, and (f) aggression, minimization of other's outcomes. However, prosocial orientation represents two specific decision rules—equality and cooperation—which tend to go hand in hand. Generally speaking, people who seek to enhance what is best for all (cooperation) also tend to value equality in outcomes (Van Lange 1999, 2006).

The typology of interpersonal orientations is primarily designed to help understand interpersonal behaviour in various situations studied by social and behavioural scientists. In particular, it has been shown to account for behaviour in various social dilemma tasks, in various negotiation tasks, and other settings rooted in experimental games (e.g. Van Lange 1999). Prosocials, who seek to enhance equality in outcomes and joint outcomes, exhibit greater cooperation in such situations than do people who seek to enhance their own outcomes in an absolute sense (individualists) or relative to others (competitors). Moreover, it has been shown to predict a wide variety of behaviours in other settings, such that relative to people with individualistic and competitive orientations, people with prosocial orientations are more likely to sacrifice in ongoing close relationships, to engage in citizenship behaviours, to volunteer in psychological experiments (with and without course credit), and to donate to help to the poor and the ill (Van Lange et al 2005). We also suggest that the interpersonal orientations should be of central relevance to various other prosocial behaviours, emotions and cognitions, such as expressions of gratitude, trust and suspicion, and spontaneous helping.

The major goal of the present paper is to review evidence in support of two interpersonal orientations: altruism and equality. That is, we seek to illustrate the relevance of these two decision rules in guiding interpersonal behaviour in various settings. We focus on these two orientations, because *empathy* is assumed to be a key determinant of altruism, and because *equality* is key component of fairness. The reader interested in the other interpersonal orientations should consult Van Lange

(1999, for a comprehensive analysis, see Van Lange et al 2006). In discussing altruism and equality, we begin by outlining some key features of a social interaction analysis to these orientations.

A social interaction analysis

What does it mean to adopt a social interaction analysis to empathy and fairness? It means at least four things. First, it means that it conceptualizes these tendencies in terms of social interactions, which are defined in terms of persons and situations (see Kelley et al 2003). Specifically, for a dyad, social interaction is defined as:

$$\text{Social Interaction} = F \text{ (Self, Partner and Situation)}$$

A key component of interaction is the Situation, as they afford various orientations that people may take to these situations. For example, a social dilemma focuses on the conflict between self-interest and collective interest, thereby affording 'selfishness' (such as the direct pursuit own outcomes) and 'cooperation' (such as the pursuit of collective outcomes). But importantly, by examining interactions, we also see that orientations such as equality become important. For example, equality as an instance of fairness may become important because of influences regarding the Self (e.g. I hold a prosocial orientation, and thus wish to pursue equality in outcomes) because of Partner influences (e.g. the Partner holds a competitive orientation by which equality becomes very salient), or because the situation represents inequality (e.g. one has greater outcomes than the other when they initiated the interaction). Similarly, altruism is also activated by the self, the partner and the situation, as there is interindividual variability in empathy (e.g. dispositional empathy, Davis 1983), empathy may be more strongly activated by some partners than by others (e.g. one's child vs. stranger), and some situational features are especially likely to call for empathy (e.g. when the partner is strongly dependent on your help).

Second, a social interaction analysis provides a fairly inclusive analysis, in that it allows us to focus on *both* distal and proximal determinants of social interactions. Examples of distal determinants are personality variables (e.g. differences in prosocial, individualistic and competitive orientations, Van Lange et al 1997), relational variables (e.g. differences in trust in the partner; differences in relational commitment; e.g. Rusbult & Van Lange 2003), and situational variables (e.g. climates of trust versus distrust; group size). Examples of proximal mechanisms (which often are both a determinant and a consequence of social interactions) are emotions (e.g. feelings of guilt, feelings of shame), and cognitions (e.g. how the situation is 'defined', especially in terms of norms and roles; Van Lange et al 2006). For example, prosocials may believe that others tend to be prosocial, individualistic or competitive, whereas competitors tend to believe that most or all others are competitive. Such beliefs may be rooted in social interaction experiences, with prosocials often developing interactions of mutual cooperation or mutual non-cooperation, and competitors often developing interactions of mutual non-cooperation. The latter experiences confirm their belief that 'all people are competitive', even though in many cases it may have been the result of their own actions: indeed, a perfect example of a self-fulfilling prophecy (Kelley & Stahelski 1970). Thus, this example shows that beliefs can affect interaction outcomes, which in turn can affect beliefs.

Third, a social interaction analysis is also important from the perspective of *observation* and *learning*. Social interactions are largely observable to the self, to the other, as well as to third parties who may not be involved (e.g. observers). As such, the manner in which social interactions unfold (e.g. two people on the route to cooperation versus two people on the route to noncooperation due to one person's lack of cooperation) serves important communicative purposes—both for the interactants and for the observers. The interactants may signal their boundaries of cooperation (e.g. by communicating threats and promises), and learn from their actions in their interactions (e.g. 'Next time, I will more carefully examine his responses to my cooperative initiatives'). Observers may learn as well, an example being children copying and 'learning from' interactions between their parents. The point is that social interaction experiences will often provide the basis for the development of a particular personality style. For example, people raised in larger families may be more likely to develop an orientation of equality because the situations that are enter are more likely to call for sharing (e.g. they learn quickly that not sharing is a dysfunctional way in which to solve social dilemmas; see Van Lange et al 1997).

Finally, a social interaction analysis dictates the importance of interpersonal orientations; that is, the preferences that people have regarding the ways in which outcomes are allocated to themselves and others. We suggest that there are six important orientations, or decision rules, that can be meaningfully distinguished: Altruism, cooperation, equality, individualism, competition and aggression. As alluded to earlier, we discuss two of these orientations in turn, namely *altruism* and *equality*.

Altruism

The claim that altruism should be considered an interpersonal orientation is rather controversial. Indeed, as most readers know, there has been a fair amount of debate about the existence of altruism both within and beyond psychology. Much of the controversy, however, deals with definitions of altruism, ranging from behavioural definitions (i.e. acts of costly helping are considered altruistic; Fehr & Gächter 2002) to definitions that seek to exclude any possible mechanism that may be activated by some consideration that may not be free of self-interest (e.g. Cialdini et al 1997). If we limit our discussion, for parsimony's sake, to research on cooperation and competition, and to allocation measures, then we see that altruism is not very prominent. For example, in assessments of interpersonal orientations in a specific resource allocation task, the percentage of people who should be classified as altruistic (i.e. assigning no weight to their own outcomes while assigning substantial weight to other's outcomes) is close to zero (Liebrand & Van Run 1985). Similarly, when people playing a single-choice prisoner's dilemma observe that the other makes a non-cooperative choice, the percentage of cooperation drops to 5% or less (Van Lange 1999).

But this evidence should not be interpreted as if altruism does not exist. In fact, what is more likely is that it does not exist under the (interpersonal) circumstances that are common in this tradition of research. People usually face a decision-making task, be it a social dilemma task, a resource allocation task, or a negotiation task, in which they are interdependent with a 'relative stranger' in that there is no history of social interaction or other form of relationship. Accordingly, there is no basis for feelings of interpersonal attachment, sympathy, or relational commitment. We suggest that when such feelings are activated, altruism may very well exist. In fact, relative strangers (even animals) can elicit empathy, as we know from some movies (e.g. the killing of Bambi's mother in *Bambi*), a point which is powerfully illustrated in research by Batson and colleagues.

As a case in point, Batson and Ahmad (2001) had participants play a single-trial prisoner's dilemma in which the other made the first choice. Before the social dilemma task, the other shared some personal information that her partner had ended the relationship with her, and that she finds it hard to think about anything else. Batson and Ahmad compared three conditions, one of which was a high-empathy condition in which participants were asked to imagine and adopt the other person's perspective. The other conditions were either a low-empathy condition, which participants were instructed to take an objective perspective on the information shared by the other, or a condition in which no personal information was shared. After these instructions, participants were informed that the other make a non-cooperative choice. Batson and Ahmad found that nearly half of the participants (45%) in the high-empathy condition made a cooperative choice, while the percentages in the other low empathy and control conditions were very low, as shown in earlier research (less than 5%, as in Van Lange 1999). Hence, this study provides a powerful demonstration of the power of empathy in activating choices that can be understood in terms of altruism, in that high-empathy participants presumably assigned substantial weight to the outcomes for the other at the expense of their own outcomes.

Recent research has also shown that in the context of iterated social dilemmas, empathy can activate generosity; that is, giving more resources to the other than one received from the other. In fact, empathy can help individuals cope better with misunderstandings because the increased generosity may be interpreted in terms of trustworthiness—an attribute that is essential for dealing with misunderstandings (Rumble et al 2005). However, empathy may not always yield benefits at the collective level. There is some research indicating that feelings of empathy could promote choices that benefit one particular individual in a group—at the expense of outcomes for the entire group (Batson et al 1995). As such, just as selfishness, empathy can sometimes form a threat to cooperative interaction. That is, feelings of empathy may lead one to provide tremendous support to one particular person, thereby neglecting the well-being of the collective. For example, as noted by Batson et al (1995, p 621), an executive may retain an ineffective employee for he or she feels compassion to the detriment of the organization.

The important point is that empathy can be a powerful motivator of choice in social dilemmas—it depends on the situation whether empathy serves the collective or not. Moreover, we suggest that tendencies toward altruism are likely to be observed when individuals deal with others with whom they have developed attachment, closeness or sympathy (for an illustration on forgiveness, see Karremans et al 2003). We speculate that, ultimately, the functional value of empathy derives from helping others in need; indeed, if we were completely unable to empathize, then our children would be less likely to survive, through important failures to help.

Egalitarianism

The existence of egalitarianism or equality may be derived from various lines of research. To begin with, several experiments have been conducted within the realm of resource-sharing tasks to examine the factors that may determine different 'rules of fairness'. In these tasks, a group of people shares a resource and the problem that these decision-makers are confronted with is how to optimally use the resource without overusing it. Research by Allison & Messick (1990) provided a powerful demonstration of what happens in such situations. That is, their results showed that when participants (in a group of six people) are asked to harvest first from the common resource, people almost without exception use the equal division rule. Individuals tend to favour equality in outcomes (rather than more complicated rules of fairness). Allison & Messick (1990) suggested that equality represents a decision heuristic that has the advantages of being simple, efficient and fair. As such, equality has great potential to promote the quality and effectiveness of interpersonal relationships, and therefore can be considered as a 'decision rule' that is deeply rooted in people's orientations toward others.

Another powerful illustration of equality in interdependence situations is when people have to negotiate allocations (e.g. how to allocate monetary outcomes). This problem is often addressed in research on ultimatum bargaining games, an exceedingly popular paradigm in experimental economics (see Güth et al 1982). In this negotiation setting, two players have to decide on how to distribute a certain amount of money. One of the players, the allocator, offers a proportion of the money to the other player, the recipient. If the recipient accepts, the money will be distributed in agreement with the allocator's offer. If the recipient rejects the offer, both players get nothing. Some of the first studies using this research paradigm demonstrated that allocators generally proposed an equal distribution (i.e. a 50–50 split) of the money (for an overview, see Camerer & Thaler 1995).

Although equality is in the eye of many the prime example of fairness, we already noted that fairness might also take different forms, independent of outcomes. More precisely, allocating outcomes is always accompanied by procedures guiding allocation decisions (Thibaut & Walker 1975). People also wonder about how fair these procedures are and these perceptions in turn have also strong effects on people's behaviours and experiences in social relationships. The focus on procedural fairness was further inspired by research showing that when people are asked to talk about their personal experiences of injustice they are usually found to talk primarily about procedural issues, in particular about being treated with a lack of dignity and politeness when dealing with others (e.g. Mikula et al 1990). Also, equality tends to be essential in predicting cognitions, feelings and behaviours that are relevant to large-scale societal problems, such as helping or protecting the environment, the poor, or the ill—presumably because 'it isn't fair' (e.g. Schultz et al 2005, Van Lange et al 2006).

To conclude, egalitarianism has received attention in distinct literatures, often supporting the notion that equality in outcomes and treatment is deeply rooted in our system, in that equality often serves as a powerful, highly internalized norm as well as a heuristic for own actions and expectations regarding others' actions. Equality is not always functional, as it may be conflicting with other prosocial trust-building activities, such as forgiveness or generosity (Van Lange et al 2002), or with tendencies to follow bad apples (non-cooperative others) rather good apples (cooperative others) in a group (Ouwerkerk et al 2005).

Concluding remarks

This chapter reviews evidence in support of the existence of two conceptually independent orientations—altruism and egalitarianism—thereby illuminating how and why these orientations may affect behaviour and interactions the way they do. Through the dominance of the assumption of 'rational self-interest' in theory and research, the orientations of altruism and equalitarianism have been seriously underappreciated (as well as cooperation, competition and aggression). As such, we think that a social interactional approach to interpersonal orientations, while inherently social psychological, cuts across several shifts in the dominant theoretical paradigms in the past as well as integrates several fields of psychology—which is arguably important for any scientific topic to grow, bloom and progress to yield cumulative knowledge (e.g. Van Lange 2006). Interpersonal orientation should shape a wide variety of specific interactions and behaviours in specific situations. The list is endlessly long, and is illustrated by (but by no means limited to) concepts such as altruism, generosity, fairness, equality, cooperation, forgiveness, sacrifice, trust, conflict, aggression, hostility, reactance, competition, suspicion, retaliation and so on. Most of these topics are essential to understanding relationships among kin, friends, close partners, or colleagues, as well as group interactions among members of teams, work units, interest groups, and even nations. A challenge for the immediate future is to integrate various levels of analyses—from basic biological processes to large-scale societal-level processes, and from analyses focusing on the individual to analyses focusing on the social environment—to fully understand interpersonal orientations and their observable manifestations in interaction situations (for illustrations, see Frith & Wopert 2004, Singer & Frith 2006). Last but not least, we should note that we hardly touched upon the societal relevance of altruism and egalitarianism—to some degree, this was a deliberative decision, as we believe that in an era of terrorism, natural disaster and misunderstanding, the broader importance of altruism (through empathy) and fairness goes without saying.

Acknowledgements

This research was supported by a grant to Paul Van Lange from the Netherlands Organization of Scientific Research (NWO; Grant No. R-57–178).

References

Allison ST, Messick DM 1990 Social decision heuristics in the use of shared resources. J Behav Decis Making 3:23–42

Batson CD, Ahmad N 2001 Empathy-induced altruism in a prisoner's dilemma II: What if the target of empathy has defected? Eur J Soc Psychol 31:25–36

Batson CD, Batson JG, Todd RM, Brummett BH, Shaw LL, Aldeguer CMR 1995 Empathy and collective good: Caring for one of the others in a social dilemma. J Pers Soc Psychol 68:619–631

Camerer C, Thaler RH 1995 Anomalies: Ultimatums, dictators and manners. J Econ Perspect 9:209–219

Cialdini RB, Brown SL, Lewis BP, Luce C, Neuberg SL 1997 Reinterpreting the empathy-altruism relationship: When one into one equals oneness. J Pers Soc Psychol 73:481–494

Davis MH 1983 The effects of dispositional empathy on emotional reactions and helping—a multidimensional approach. J Pers 51:167–184

Fehr E, Gächter S 2002 Altruistic punishment in humans. Nature 415:137–140

Frith C, Wolpert D 2004 The neuroscience of social interaction: Decoding, imitating, and influencing the actions of others. Oxford University Press, Oxford

Güth W, Schmittberger R, Schwarze B 1982 An experimental analysis of ultimatum games. Econ Behav Organ 3:367–388

Karremans JC, Van Lange PAM, Ouwerkerk JW, Kluwer ES 2003 When forgiving enhances psychological well-being: The role of interpersonal commitment. J Pers Soc Psychol 84: 1011–1026

Kelley HH, Stahelski AJ 1970 Social interaction basis of cooperators' and competitors' beliefs about others. J Pers Soc Psychol 16:66–91

Kelley HH, Thibaut JW 1978 Interpersonal relations: A theory of interdependence. Wiley, New York

Kelley HH, Holmes JW, Kerr NL, Reis HT, Rusbult CE, Van Lange PAM 2003 An atlas of interpersonal situations. Cambridge University Press, New York

Liebrand WBG, Van Run GJ 1985 The effects of social motives on behavior in social dilemmas in two cultures. J Exp Soc Psychol 21:86–102

Mikula G, Petri B, Tanzer NK 1990 What people regard as unjust: Types and structures of everyday experiences of injustice. Eur J Soc Psychol 20:133–149

Miller DT 1999 The norm of self-interest. Am Psychol 54:1053–1060

Ouwerkerk JW, Kerr NL, Gallucci M, Van Lange PAM 2005 Avoiding the social death penalty: Ostracism and cooperation in social dilemmas. In: Williams KD, Forgas JP, von Hippel W (eds) The social outcast: Ostracism, social exclusion, rejection, and bullying. Psychology Press, New York, p 321–332

Rumble AC, Van Lange PAM, Parks CD 2005 The benefits of empathy: When empathy may sustain cooperation in social dilemmas. Ohio State University, unpublished manuscript

Rusbult CE, Van Lange PA 2003 Interdependence, interaction, and relationships. Annu Rev Psychol 54:351–375

Schultz PW, Gouveia VV, Cameron LD, Tankha G, Schmuck P, Franek M 2005 Values and their relationship to environmental concern and conservation behavior. J Cross Cult Psychol 36:457–475

Singer T, Frith CD 2006 The emergence of the 'social' in cognitive neuroscience: The study of interacting brains. In: Van Lange PAM (ed), Bridging social psychology: Benefits of transdisciplinary approaches. Erlbaum, Mahwah, NJ p97–102

Thibaut JW, Walker L 1975 Procedural justice: A psychological analysis. Erlbaum, Hillsdale, NJ

Van Lange PAM 1999 The pursuit of joint outcomes and equality in outcomes: An integrative model of social value orientation. J Pers Soc Psychol 77:337–349

Van Lange PAM (ed) 2006 Bridging social psychology: Benefits of transdisciplinary approaches. Erlbaum, Mahwah, NJ

Van Lange PAM, Sedikides C 1998 Being more honest but not necessarily more intelligent than others: Generality and explanations for The Muhammad Ali effect. Eur J Soc Psychol 28:675–680

Van Lange PAM, Otten W, De Bruin ENM, Joireman JA 1997 Development of prosocial, individualistic, and competitive orientations: Theory and preliminary evidence. J Pers Soc Psychol 73:733–746

Van Lange PAM, Ouwerkerk JW, Tazelaar MJA 2002 How to overcome the detrimental effects of noise in social interaction: The benefits of generosity. J Pers Soc Psychol 82:768–780

Van Lange PAM, De Cremer D, Van Dijk E, Van Vugt M 2006 Self-interest and beyond: The psychology of interpersonal orientations. In: Higgins ET, Kruglanksi AW (eds), Social psychology: Handbook of basic principles. Guilford Press, New York, in press

DISCUSSION

Gergely: Have you looked at factors such as religiosity? Does religiosity modulate this strategy?

Van Lange: There is a small link that is not too great in terms of effect size. It works more for some religions more than others. It did not account for the age effect, for example, because people of some religions may have larger families.

Gergely: Have you applied your work to in-group/out-group contexts?

Van Lange: The in-group/out-group context is interesting. I would claim that a lot of orientations, such as empathy, can be dysfunctional for some other good cause, such as collective well being. For example, sometimes people are so cooperative to their in-group that this is detrimental to the larger collective. Wars can be explained by this. Cooperation can have bad consequences when you have multi-level social environment, with in-groups and out-groups. I also think that often problems arise because you can't compare many things. There are many things that people put in the equality formula that complicate things, especially in an inter-group context. A stable finding in the social dilemma literature is when you look at interactions between individuals and interactions between three-person groups, the groups are much more competitive with one another than individuals are. Individuals are fairly trustful of one another, but groups are very distrustful of one another.

Singer: If you correlate social value orientation with classic empathy scales do you find a positive correlation between these two measures?

Van Lange: We haven't done that yet. We have looked at other measures, and there is a link between social value orientation and self report of trust. Competitors have low trust, whereas individualists, especially prosaically have higher trust. Competitors really think that the world consists of competitors, and for them it makes sense to compete even when the situation doesn't call for it. Also, when you think about competition it is often a tendency driven not so much by the desire to win, but by aversion to getting less than others. This is a very strong aversion in competitors. They would do almost anything to ensure that they do not get less than others.

Singer: How did Batson induce empathy to measure how empathy can prime prosocial behaviour? Did you used such priming techniques yourself and observe how this affects prosocial behaviour on your scales?

Van Lange: Batson used two instructions. First, subjects listened to a story about someone else. The person is asked to write a story about something that has happened. This person says they would like to write a nice story, but the only thing they can think of now is that they have been dumped the previous weekend, so it is a sad story. Then Batson used two instructions. One is to take an objective point of view, and the second is to think of what it means to be the other person. The latter empathy instruction induces empathy and in turn altruism. He has done lots of experiments that make it at least plausible that there is a link between empathy and true altruism. I recently did a study in which I used these instructions. I had a very sad story about a father who was diagnosed with cancer, and the instruction didn't matter at all but this manipulation was really powerful. When people are in an empathy mode they behave prosocially without any instrumental reason. We compared a dictator game with an ultimatum bargaining game. In the dictator game you see high levels of cooperation among those who have high levels of empathy. The work suggests that empathy can be automatically activated, without an instruction, and exert strong influences on altruistic motivation and behaviour.

Brosnan: Some of the research that I have done with monkeys indicates that the ones that are more interested in fairness may show this preference in their own self interest. They are fair, in the sense of paying attention to the other's outcomes, when it makes a difference to their own outcome (Brosnan et al 2006). How do you distinguish this from a competitive situation? I would say it is being rather competitive if you are only fair because it will increase your outcome in the end.

Van Lange: Competitors wouldn't stop. Once they get more, they just continue.

Brosnan: In this case they got relatively more rewards than their partner, both overall and of just high-value rewards, if they behaved 'unfairly', but they got absolutely more, again both overall and of high-value rewards, over the long term by being fair, because their partners quit participating if they were unfair and then neither monkey got anything at all.

Van Lange: Competitors go for relative gain over others. Even if they have bad outcomes, as long as the others do worse the competitors are happy. And they cannot stand getting just a little less than others.

Silk: I wanted to go back to the point about whether these prosocial orientations might have an adaptive value. Have you any information about the relationship between prosocial orientation and something that would give a measure of quality of social life, such as size of social network or numbers of friends?

Van Lange: We need to look at this. I once asked these questions and got a lot of variation in terms of, for example, the number of friends that people report. People use different definitions of friends. The relationship that they have with their parents can be very important for the development of social value orientations. There is a link between social value orientation and attachment. It is the aspect of attachment that has to do with trust, showing that competitors have low trust and are the least likely to be securely attached.

Silk: There is a lot of literature suggesting that the quality of people's social networks has very important effects on health. My intuitive model would be that prosocial people might be better at maintaining social relationships. The bit of data you cited as evidence against this, that prosocial orientation declines after 65, is not a good argument against this hypothesis. Selection is weak at these old ages because people at these ages are no longer reproducing. Natural selection is not as strong on traits that are expressed in old age.

Van Lange: If there is a link between quality of life and prosocial orientation, it is a linear link. It would be the case that individualists and competitors die earlier. After 65 you would have a drop in these traits in the population. I strongly believe in the functionality of prosocial orientation. I started a programme of research on studying the benefits of generosity, generosity being defined as doing just a little bit more than the other did (Van Lange et al 2002). In the coin paradigm, you can compare a strict tit-for-tat strategy with a tit-for-tat-plus-one strategy. In the latter, the subject always gives one coin more than they have received. In normal situations they do equally well, but when there is noise, a basis of misunderstanding, then tit-for-tat-plus-one does better.

Blair: From what you were saying in answer to the in-group/out-group question it looked like you were suggesting that there was a big difference between in-group/out-group. However, in your data the big real world correlate was with out-group giving. It looked like your prosocials were pretty in-group and out-group focused relative to the other two conditions.

Van Lange: That is the kind of situation where the in-group/out-group distinctions were not salient. You can study two distinct groups and examine how they act in an interdependent situation toward one another. In the paradigm I just described we have groups of three people and they make a decision in a prisoner's dilemma. Then we see there is very little cooperation between the two groups.

Blair: The distinction is between the prosocial individuals versus the competitive individuals. If you had a three person group of prosocials versus a three person group of competitors, surely you would predict that the group of prosocials would be less competitive? Otherwise you are putting two different things together: predisposition at the individual level and what happens when you join people together in groups.

Van Lange: Often people believe that empathy, cooperation and fairness are always 'good' for the group or collective. This is frequently the case, but they can have drawbacks. I am probably referring more to the exceptions rather than the rules. Empathy has a drawback that you could be partial, benefiting one person over others, which can have bad consequences for an organization, for example. This may be a limitation of empathy and altruism. The same is true for cooperation. There are situations where if you only think in terms of your in-group cooperation this may not be a functional attitude. It can have bad consequences. With fairness, if people are always good at book keeping and don't think of exchange possibilities in the future, this will also be detrimental to future exchange. If you always do tit-for-tat immediately you can run into problems.

U Frith: You have talked about many different factors and situations that might influence these social value orientations. But one I missed is status. I think an interaction with status could explain a lot of the results that you described. For example, if you are a generous person, you are immediately asserting that you might be able to afford to give because you have more than the other. Age could also be a factor. As you get older, on the whole you are getting wealthier and you should become more prosocial and generous. No doubt, as you get even older, the situation reverses. I have a general question: if you had a big discrepancy in age and status, such as a small child who has nothing and a powerful adult, who has everything, and you saw evidence of empathy in the child towards the adult, what would you experience, and what would this tell us? I think it would be an extremely powerful effect, much more so than the adult showing empathy to the child.

Van Lange: There is a whole literature about this. When you are in a superior position you should give more. It is an established norm in social responsibility that if you can give and you are in a situation to do it, you should do this. You should offer help if you can. This could also underlie the findings of the donations. I agree with you: I would probably discuss this under the heading of normative influences.

Montague: I missed something. Were there other metrics along which you categorized these prosocial people, or did you just use your three-category task?

Van Lange: We used variations of that task.

Montague: In that task I have three choices, and there are differences along the other axes, but in the middle choice there are two variables that change. If I was going to consider these, I would put people in a forced-choice paradigm, but it is an unfair comparison to compare two variables in the middle choice.

Van Lange: This is a nine-item version based on many different methods. There are also more elaborate 36-item versions. There is often a strong correspondence between those methods, in that they yield similar findings. For example, independent of the instrument for assessing social value orientation, you will see that prosocials behave more cooperatively than do individualists and competitors, that they respond differently to others pursuing tit-for-tat strategies, and so on. Therefore, I have started to use the nine-item version, which predicts as well as the other, longer versions.

Montague: My intuition is as follows. There is nothing social about that task. I don't see you probing anything social. This is why it is remarkable that when you do these other metrics this very calculating division across these choices co-varies with all these things we consider as prosocial behaviour. This is why I was interested in the comment about the Machiavellian view that I am doing some sort of externalized display of status or desired status, and somehow that elevates me.

Moll: I have a question about sensitivity to injustice. There is a study (Schmitt & Mohiyeddini 1996) showing that prosocials tend to be less sensitive to injustice towards themselves and more to injustice to others. Do you see this?

Van Lange: I think the prosocials are quite concerned with equality for themselves also.

Moll: Have you tested this in your studies?

Van Lange: I don't know of any evidence on this. I agree. It would be interesting to examine how prosocials respond to violations of justice that does or does not involve themselves.

Moll: There is some evidence that if people believe more in a just world they tend to be less annoyed by injustice to themselves (Schmitt & Mohiyeddini 1996).

Silk: The remark about status entering into it is one of the predominant models in evolutionary psychology about why people are so cooperative. It is a version of what is called the costly signalling model in biology. It costs more for a poor person to give things away than it does for a rich person. The problem with applying this model as a deep explanation for this behaviour is that there is no reason why the signal of giving money away to other people should be valued. Why don't rich people just burn it? Why wouldn't we admire that? The question is, why is it that we value the prosocial demonstration of wealth rather than just conspicuous consumption?

References

Brosnan SF, Freeman C, de Waal FB 2006 Partner's behavior, not reward distribution, determines success in an unequal cooperative task in capuchin monkeys. Am J Primatol 68:713–724

Schmitt M, Mohiyeddini C 1996 Sensitivity to befallen injustice and reactions to a real-life disadvantage. Social Justice Res 9:223–238

Van Lange PAM, Ouwerkerk J, Tazelaar M 2002 How to overcome the detrimental effects of noise in social interaction: the benefits of generosity. J Personal Social Psychol 82:768–780

Triggering the intentional stance

Raymond A. Mar and C. Neil Macrae*[1]

*Department of Psychology, University of Toronto, 100 St. George Street, Toronto, ON M5S 3G3, Canada, and *School of Psychology, University of Aberdeen, King's College, Aberdeen AB24 2UB, UK*

Abstract. While humans possess a ready capacity to view a target (biological or otherwise) as an intentional agent (i.e. the 'intentional stance'), the conditions necessary for spontaneously eliciting these mentalizing processes are less well understood. Although research examining people's tendency to construe the motion of geometric shapes as intentional has done much to illuminate this issue, due to methodological limitations (a reliance on subjective self-report) this work has not fully addressed the potentially automatic and obligatory nature of mentalizing. Acknowledging this problem, recent research using prelinguistic infants, neuroimaging technology and methods that avoid explicit self-report all provide unique paths to circumvent this shortcoming. While work of this kind has generally corroborated the results of previous investigations, it has also raised a number of new issues. One such issue is whether spontaneous mentalizing processes for abstract non-biological stimuli are instantiated in the same neural architecture as those for realistic representations of intentional biological agents. This question is considered in the current chapter.

2006 Empathy and Fairness. Wiley, Chichester (Novartis Foundation Symposium 278) p 111–133

Spontaneous social perception versus controlled social judgements

The ability to comprehend the beliefs, emotions and intentions of others is both characteristic of, and necessary for, successful human interaction. Our richly social nature and complex societal hierarchies demand these skills, such that those who exhibit deficits in this domain experience considerable difficulty interacting with others (e.g. individuals with autism; Tager-Flusberg 2001). Known as possessing a theory-of-mind (ToM), mentalizing, or adopting the intentional stance, this capacity to view others as possessing mental states can be directed to targets other than conspecifics. Not only are we tempted to believe that a pet hamster is 'just like a little person,' we routinely view quite abstract nonliving representations as if they were intentional agents. Be it an animated movie populated by talking

---

[1] This paper was presented at the symposium by Neil Macrae to whom correspondence should be addressed

animals, the Sunday morning cartoon strip, or a novel whose characters are represented by mere words on a page, our enjoyment of all these media depend upon
an ability to adopt the intentional stance toward clearly nonintentional (and non
biological) objects (Mar 2004, Mar et al 2006). Moreover, such engagements do
not appear to be cognitively taxing. The ease with which we can comprehend the
sorry misadventures of poor old Charlie Brown in a *Peanuts* comic strip contributes
to our enjoyment. In some cases, it certainly feels as if we cannot help but view a
representation as intentional (e.g. characters in an animated film), although we
certainly know that this perceived or felt agency is entirely illusory. Thus, while
we are capable of making social judgements when prompted, we also appear to
spontaneously and automatically perceive certain displays as representing intentional agents.

Isolating the specific qualities that evoke this illusion of intentionality has been
the subject of active research for at least half a century (Heider & Simmel 1944)
and this phenomenon has been distinguished as a form of social perception rather
than social judgement (Allison et al 2000, Scholl & Tremoulet 2000). These two
ideas—that of automatic and spontaneous perceptions of intentionality in contrast
to effortful and controlled judgements of the same—appears to parallel a number
of theoretical splits within the literature on mentalizing. Explanations for ToM
have tended to group around two competing general ideas: theory-theory and
simulation-theory (Carruthers & Smith 1996). The unfortunately named theory-
theory proposes that mentalizing is achieved through propositional, rule-based
thinking. Humans are viewed as amateur scientists with folk-psychological theories regarding the relation between mental states and behaviours, from which
predictions are made. Developmental progress in attaining a ToM, then, is seen as
the gradual construction of more accurate theories, wrought through experience
in a complex social world.

Simulation-theory, in contrast, proposes that inferring the emotions and goals
of other agents is achieved by imagining what our own feelings and aims would
be were we placed in a similar situation—by simulating the experience of this other
person. This viewpoint can be seen as resting on a form of embodied cognition,
in which the understanding of an other is built upon concurrent engagement
of affective and motor systems in the self (see Blakemore & Frith 2005, Keysars
& Perrett 2004). These two explanations are not mutually exclusive, and many
researchers are beginning to propose theories that blend the two approaches
(Carruthers & Smith 1996). Simulation-theory and theory-theory also appear part
of a broader debate concerning the existence of both a cognitive, language-based
and propositional form of mental inference (more akin to theory-theory) as well
as an emotional and embodied form of empathic understanding (in keeping with
simulation theory—Tager-Flusberg 2001, Preston & de Waal 2002). To be clear,
we are by no means putting forth the argument that social perception should be

equated with simulation-theory, nor with emotional empathy for that matter. Spontaneous mentalizing, however, can be seen as a fundamental contributing process for these broader categories. Answering questions regarding the former is absolutely necessary for understanding the latter. What are the conditions under which social perceivers spontaneously view others as intentional agents? Put differently, what triggers the adoption of the intentional stance?

Spontaneous adult mentalizing and subjective self report

Similar to how Michotte (1946/1963) revealed spontaneous perceptions of causality using very simplistic animations of moving shapes, Heider and Simmel (1944) demonstrated that inferences of intentionality can be drawn from quite abstract, non-biological representations. These researchers presented a series of short animations, each involving two triangles (one large, one small) and a circle, all moving around an empty rectangle. Observers readily attributed personality traits to the shapes and described their movements in terms of mental states such as goals and emotions, a finding replicated by subsequent researchers (for a review see Scholl & Tremoulet 2000). In general, this work has supported the idea that it is the spatiotemporal characteristics of the animations that trigger animacy descriptions (such as changes in path, moving in response to other objects and self-propelled movement) and not the featural properties of the interacting shapes (Scholl & Tremoulet 2000).

Animacy, however, while likely a necessary cue for intentionality, is not an equivalent construct (for a discussion see Gergely et al 1995). Furthermore, there are concerns about whether this method truly addresses the spontaneous and perceptual quality of these inferences. Observers report their subjective percepts in response to the animations, and it is possible that higher-order cognitive processing is engaged in order to produce these descriptions (cf. Scholl & Tremoulet 2000). Individuals may not be perceiving intentionality, but merely reporting the observation of intentional behaviour as a result of other factors such as demand characteristics and calculated inference. Thankfully, there are ways to circumvent this problem, such as employing: (1) designs that do not require explicit prompts for judgement; (2) prelinguistic infants as participants; and (3) neuroimaging approaches.

Spontaneous mentalizing in infants

Infant participants are unique in that their responses are relatively uncontaminated by cultural experience, experimental demands and language-based cognition, making them ideal subjects for examining the question of automatic social perception (Johnson 2000). Naturally, prelinguistic infants cannot self-report their percepts of intentionality while viewing animations—precluding explicit prompts for judgement—so researchers must capitalize upon their tendency to attend longer to novel displays. After an infant has been habituated to a certain visual stimulus, new displays can be shown and if they are perceived to be different from the earlier stimulus, infants will tend to look longer (see Johnson 2000, Box 1). Gergely and colleagues (1995), for example, found that 12-month old babies were more surprised and attended longer when a moving shape behaved in a seemingly non-rational manner as opposed to when it moved in a rational and goal-based fashion, even if the latter display was more perceptually dissimilar to the habituation stimulus. This finding appears to demonstrate that even prelinguistic infants attribute intentionality to abstract shapes based solely upon spatiotemporal variables. Similarly, Luo and Baillargeon (2005) have convincingly demonstrated that infants as young as 5 months old readily attribute goals to novel non-human objects (such as a box), provided that it possesses a cue of agency, such as self-propelled movement. Other evidence, however, indicates that featural properties are also important. Infants are more likely to imitate the failed goal-attempts of an adult over those of robotic pincers, are more likely to view the grasping actions of a hand as goal-directed compared to a perceptually similar rod and are more likely to follow the 'gaze' of a novel object when it has a face (for reviews see Johnson 2000, 2003). Similarly, Guajardo & Woodward (2004) have shown that infants view a bare-handed grasp as goal-directed, but do not appear to do so when this hand is covered by a glove. Importantly, when the infants had an opportunity to associate this gloved hand with a human agent, they were more likely to then attribute the grasping actions as intentional.

Johnson (2003) has reviewed the cues that are thought to trigger the intentional stance, including: (1) facial features; (2) an asymmetry along one axis; (3) non-rigid transformations such as expansion and contraction; (4) self-propelled movement; and (5) the capacity for reciprocal and contingent behaviour. It remains unclear, however, which of these cues are either necessary and/or sufficient. We are unlikely to view all objects with an asymmetry as intentional, for example, and many objects that possess the property of self-propulsion are not viewed as intentional. Her own work has shown that morphological cues (such as those possessed by a mechanical orangutan) and movement cues (such as a furry blob that behaves contingently in response to an experimenter), either individually or in combination, can signal to infants the presence of an intentional, and not just animate, agent (Johnson 2003). There are questions, of course, as to whether these behaviours by infants reflect mentalizing processes identical to those undertaken by adults. Gergely and colleagues (e.g. Gergely & Csibra 2003), for example, have argued that studies such as those reviewed above are evidence for a non-mentalistic 'teleological stance' on the part of infants, that acts as a precursor to the mentalistic intentional stance adopted by older children and adults.

Neuroimaging and the intentional stance

One of the greatest strengths of neuroimaging approaches such as functional magnetic resonance imaging (fMRI) and positron emission tomography (PET) is its potential to covertly examine mental processes without the confound of explicit probes for self-report. There have been a handful of studies that have examined the neural correlates of intentionality cues, using animations like those created by Heider and Simmel (1944). Castelli and colleagues (2000) presented three types of animations while collecting PET scans, shapes that moved: (1) randomly; (2) in a goal-directed way; and (3) in ways that implied complex mental states (such as deception). In half the cases, participants were told what sort of animation they would see (the cued condition), and the order of these blocks was counterbalanced. For half the participants then, the uncued condition followed the cued, allowing for the possibility that awareness of the animation-types biased their attention and inferences during the former condition. This may explain why no differences were found during cued and uncued animations, prompting the researchers to combine the data across conditions for analysis.

Animations meant to elicit theory-of-mind attributions elicited more activation in several areas relative to the random animations: (1) the bilateral temporal parietal junction (TPJ); in the posterior superior temporal sulcus (STS); (2) bilateral basal temporal regions, including the temporal poles; (3) the bilateral extrastriate cortex: and (4) the medial prefrontal cortex (MPFC). A follow-up study involving both autistic patients and normally developing controls replicated this finding, and also found that autistics had less activation in the basal temporal area, the STS and TPJ, and the MPFC (Castelli et al 2002). Behavioural data have shown that those with autism are less likely to report percepts of intentionality when viewing these types of stimuli, allowing for the inference that these brain areas are responsible for engaging the intentional stance (Abell et al 2000, Castelli et al 2002). Corroborating this supposition, the TPJ and STS, temporal poles and MPFC have all been implicated in mentalising processes in numerous studies, using a variety of methods and tasks (Gallagher & Frith 2003).

Blakemore and colleagues (2003) performed an influential fMRI study that employed simple shape animations to parse perceptions of animacy and contingency, as well as examine the effect of drawing attention to the contingency relations (via an explicit probe). Different parts of the brain were associated with viewing animate compared to contingent stimuli, and when both qualities were present activation was observed in superior parietal areas. Notably, when participants were cued to attend to the contingent movements, activation was observed in the right middle frontal gyrus (MFG) and left STS. It is worth noting that the stimuli in this study were much less complex than those in the previous studies, and did not involve imbuing shapes with complicated mental states.

Similar areas of activation were found in a study by Shultz and colleagues (2004), who presented animations of one circle chasing another. In half the animations, the chasing circle predicted the end-state of the other circle in order to catch it, and in the other half this circle merely followed the other. When comparing the predicting condition to the following condition, activations were observed around the STS in both hemispheres. In conjunction, similar to the findings of Blakemore and colleagues (2003), explicitly drawing attention to the 'strategy' of the circle was associated with the left STS. The STS and TPJ have proven very important for the discussion of basic cues for intentionality; a number of researchers have argued that the STS is implicated in the understanding of biological motion, specifically with respect to intentions and goals (e.g. Allison et al 2000, Pelphrey et al 2004a, Saxe et al 2004).

One question that arises from the work reviewed thus far is whether the STS also codes for featural cues that trigger the intentional stance, along with motion cues. There is some evidence for this. Activation in the STS has been observed for static images of features that cue intentionality, such as eyes, mouths, hands and faces; in some cases, however, these static images may have implied motion (for a review see Allison et al 2000). Because activations in this area are observed both when abstract shapes and realistic portrayals of biological agents are used as stimuli, it has been conjectured that the STS codes for intentional movement regardless of form (Shultz et al 2004). Direct comparisons of cartoon and realistic motion, however, are methodologically difficult to achieve. Pelphrey and colleagues (2003) found that the STS did not appear to respond differentially to the movements of a computer-animated person compared to a similarly rendered 'robot' constructed of cylinders and spheres. In contrast, a separate fMRI study found that although the STS responded to very abstract representations of biological motion (point-light displays), it demonstrated a slightly stronger response to videos of real people in motion (Beauchamp et al 2003). A PET study, involving observations of grasping actions by a real hand compared to a 3D virtual reality hand, found the right TPJ near the posterior STS was more activated by the real hand; the right temporal pole also showed a similar preference (Perani et al 2001).

In a recent study (Mar et al 2006), we examined whether the brain responds differently to complex dynamic videos of social interactions presented in either a cartoon or realistic fashion. Footage for the film *Waking Life* (Linklater 2001) was shot using real actors, and later transformed by computer animators into a cartoon. Motion kinematics from the real footage were thus preserved in the animated version, and although both versions had numerous cues for animacy and intentionality (e.g. self-propelled movement, faces and other biological features) one was obviously realistic while the other was a cartoon (see Fig. 1). Equivalent content was shown in both versions, and shots within scenes alternated between cartoon and real. Participants were not prompted to make any social judgement,

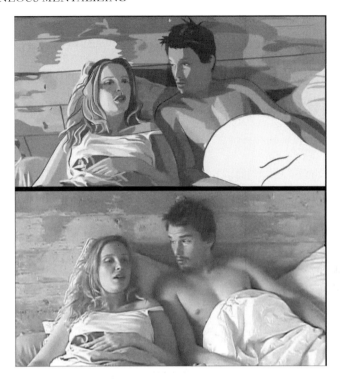

FIG. 1.   Screenshot from the video stimuli employed by Mar et al (2006); cartoon version
above real version.

but only instructed to watch the videos closely, which were presented without
sound. We found that the right STS and TPJ were more activated while participants
watched realistic scenes compared to cartoon scenes (see Fig. 2A). Even though
the cartoon version was closely matched to the real version, the latter appears to
have preferentially engaged brain areas known to be involved in mentalizing and
the inference of intentions from behaviour.

Interestingly, the right MFG was also more activated during the real condition
(see Fig. 2B), and others have found similar activations to be associated with
attending to contingency relations in the presence of animacy (Blakemore et al
2003), making judgements regarding persons (Mason et al 2004) and inferences
of intentionality when perceiving actions (Pelphrey et al 2004a). Moreover, because
this study did not employ explicit prompts for social judgement, this appears to
be evidence for the spontaneous triggering of the intentional stance based upon
perceptual cues (cf. German et al 2004). The right STS, TPJ and MFG thus appear
to be highly sensitive to subtle cues signalling intentionality, moving beyond

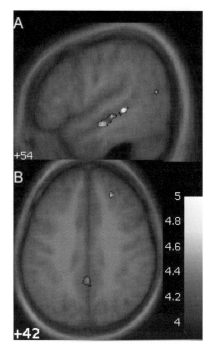

FIG. 2.   Activation in the right STS, TPJ (A) and MFG (B) for the Real > Cartoon contrast
from Mar et al (2006). Activations superimposed on an average of all T1-weighted structural
scans for participants. Legend indicates t-value.

animate motion and biological features (present in both versions of the stimuli)
to the perception of targets as belonging to the real world. Previous work has also
demonstrated such sensitivity to subtle cues of intentionality in the STS, such as
a preference for mutual gaze as opposed to averted gaze from a dynamic computer-
animated person (Pelphrey et al 2004b). It appears that activation in the STS and
TPJ may be modulated by the number of cues present that signal intentionality.
While basic motion cues (e.g. animated shapes) as well as static featural cues (e.g.
faces and eyes) can result in engagement of these superior lateral temporal regions,
combining these cues appears to result in greater activity.

Conclusions

The ability to infer intentions from the behaviours of others is clearly important
(Baldwin & Baird 2001). By understanding the basic cues that cause us to treat
a target as intentional, we can begin to explore the very foundations of social
cognition. From one perspective, our tendency to innately, automatically, and

spontaneously view a broad variety of different targets as holding goals and mental states seems to fly in the face of parsimony and pragmatism. Why can our intentional stance be triggered so easily, and by so many stimuli that are clearly *not* intentional? How useful is a system when it often renders conclusions that do not reflect reality? We have no clear way of knowing that other agents, even other humans, are truly intentional (i.e. the solipsistic conundrum). Therefore, it may be that a low threshold for triggering the intentional stance—a bias toward viewing agents as having goals, beliefs, and desires—provides us with an adaptive heuristic for understanding our world and all its inhabitants.

Acknowledgements

The writing of this chapter was supported in part by a Social Sciences and Humanities Research Council of Canada fellowship to RAM.

References

Abell F, Happé F, Frith U 2000 Do triangles play tricks? Attribution of mental states to animated shapes in normal and abnormal development. Cognitive Devt 15:1–16

Allison T, Puce A, McCarthy G 2000 Social perception from visual cues: role of the STS region. Trends Cogn Sci 4:267–278

Baldwin DA, Baird JA 2001 Discerning intentions in dynamic human interaction. Trends Cogn Sci 5:171–178

Beauchamp MS, Lee KE, Haxby JV, Martin A 2003 fMRI response to video and point-light displays of moving humans and manipulable objects. J Cognitive Neurosci 15:991–1001

Blakemore S-J, Frith C 2005 The role of motor contagion in the prediction of action. Neuropsychologia 43:260–267

Blakemore S-J, Boyer P, Pachot-Clouard M, Segebarth C, Decety J 2003 The detection of contingency and animacy from simple animations in the human brain. Cereb Cortex 13: 837–844

Carruthers P, Smith PK (eds) 1996 Theories of theories of mind. Cambridge University Press, Cambridge, MA

Castelli F, Happé F, Frith U, Frith C 2000 Movement and mind: a functional imaging study of perception and interpretation of complex intentional movement patterns. NeuroImage 12: 314–325

Castelli F, Frith C, Happé F, Frith U 2002 Autism, Asperger syndrome and brain mechanisms for the attribution of mental states to animated shapes. Brain 125:1839–1849

Dennet D 1987 The intentional stance. MIT Press, Cambridge, MA

Gallagher HL, Frith CD 2003 Functional imaging of 'theory of mind'. Trends Cogn Sci 7: 77–83

Gergely G, Csibra G 2003 Teleological reasoning in infancy: the naïve theory of rational action. Trends Cogn Sci 7:287–292

Gergely G, Nádasy Z, Csibra G, Bíró S 1995 Taking the intentional stance at 12 months of age. Cognition 56:165–193

German TP, Niehaus JL, Roarty MP, Giesbrecht B, Miller MB 2004 Neural correlates of detecting pretense: Automatic engagement of the intentional stance under covert conditions. J Cognitive Neurosci 16:1805–1817

Guajardo JJ, Woodward AL 2004 Is agency skin deep? Surface attributes influence infants' sensitivity to goal-directed action. Infancy 6:361–384

Heider F, Simmel M 1944 An experimental study of apparent behavior. Am J Psychol 57: 243–249

Johnson SC 2000 The recognition of mentalistic agents in infancy. Trends Cogn Sci 4:22–28

Johnson SC 2003 Detecting agents. Philos Trans R Soc Lond B Biol Sci, Series B, 358: 549–559

Keysars C, Perrett DI 2004 Demystifying social cognition: a Hebbian perspective. Trends Cogn Sci 8:501–507

Linklater R 2001 Waking Life. Fox Searchlight Pictures, Los Angeles

Luo Y, Baillargeon R 2005 Can a self-propelled box have a goal? Psychol Sci 16:601–608

Mar RA 2004 The neuropsychology of narrative: story comprehension, story production and their interrelation. Neuropsychologia 42:1414–1434

Mar RA, Kelley WM, Heatherton TF, Macrae CN 2006 Detecting agency from biological motion, in preparation

Mar RA, Oatley K, Hirsh J, dela Paz J, Peterson JB 2006 Bookworms versus nerds: Exposure to fiction versus non-fiction, divergent associations with social ability, and the simulation of fictional worlds. J Res Pers, in press

Mason MF, Banfield JF, Macrae CN 2004 Thinking about actions: The neural substrates of person knowledge. Cereb Cortex 14:209–214

Michotte A 1946/English Trans 1963 The perception of causality. Basic Books, New York

Pelphrey KA, Mitchell TV, McKeown MJ, Goldstein J, Allison T, McCarthy G 2003 Brain activity evoked by the perception of human walking: Controlling for meaningful coherent action. J Neurosci 23:6819–6825

Pelphrey KA, Morris JP, McCarthy G 2004a Grasping the intentions of others: The perceived intentionality of an action influences the activity in the superior temporal sulcus during social perception. J Cognitive Neurosci 16:1706–1716

Pelphrey KA, Viola RJ, McCarthy G 2004b When strangers pass: Processing of mutual and averted social gaze in the superior temporal sulcus. Psychol Sci 15:598–603

Perani D, Fazio F, Borghese NA et al 2001 Different brain correlates for watching real and virtual hand actions. NeuroImage 14:749–758

Preston SD, de Waal FBM 2002 Empathy: Its ultimate and proximate bases. Behav Brain Sci 25:1–20

Saxe R, Xiao D-K, Kovacs G, Perrett DI, Kanwisher N 2004 A region of right posterior superior temporal sulcus responds to observed intentional actions. Neuropsychologia 42:1435–1446

Scholl BJ, Tremoulet PD 2000 Perceptual causality and animacy. Trends Cogn Sci 4:299–309

Shultz J, Imamizu H, Kawato M, Frith CD 2004 Activation of human superior temporal gyrus during observation of goal attribution by intentional objects. J Cognitive Neurosci 16: 1695–1705

Tager-Flusberg H 2001 A re-examination of the theory-of-mind hypothesis of autism. In: Burack J, Charman T, Yimiya N, Zelazo P (eds) The development of autism: Perspectives from theory and research. Lawrence Erlbaum Associates, Mahwah, NJ p 173–193

DISCUSSION

C Frith: It might be useful for us to discuss the uncanny valley. It is a concept developed in Japan and relates to animation. This is supposed to explain why some recent animated films didn't work. Animations are getting better and better in terms of their realism, and as they become more human-like they elicit responses from viewers that are more positive and empathic. But there is a point of increased realism at which they become uncanny, and people find them repulsive. This is the uncanny valley. Our colleague Thierry Chaminade has looked at this specifically. He took point light walkers, which were originally made by putting light sources on nine joints of a person and then filming them walking along in the dark. Even though all you see is the spots of light you can instantly recognise that it is a person walking. Then you can dress the light spots up as Godzilla or a robot or a person, producing interesting effects. The point light walker is described as having the most realistic motion even though the motion is in fact identical in these three cases. The more you make the figure realistic the more you are aware that the movement is not quite right. This is an interesting observation. There are now all sorts of ways of doing this kind of experiment, using 3D animation software where you can capture the movement and turn it into a cartoon. You were making the point that this interesting relationship between the self and the other is because our primitive mechanisms for understanding ourselves can then be applied to understanding other people. I would like to suggest that it is actually the other way round: the important thing in life is to learn how to explain the behaviour of other people. We find we can do this rather efficiently by thinking about their mental states. Then perhaps we are able to apply that to ourselves, otherwise what is the point of thinking of our own mental states?

U Frith: Is the understanding of ourselves and of others an automatic and unconscious process or do we need to reflect on it?

Gallese: There is a lot of research done in social psychology showing that people don't know what they want. They rationalize after the act.

Macrae: In terms of your own writings on decoupling beliefs from reality (I guess developmental psychologists would have a story to tell here), would that originate in decoupling self beliefs from self-experienced reality and knowing that you can be entertaining things in your head that bear no resemblance to the contexts or situations that you find yourself in? Perhaps self is the generator and not the other.

C Frith: It is not clear whether you need to have self before the other. Francesca Happé, for example, has claimed that it is the other way round with inferences about the mental states of others coming before inferences about mental states of the self (Happé 2003).

U Frith: I want to remind you of the Alan Leslie's story. He originally conceptualized decoupling as the critical mechanism in mentalizing. You need to be able to quarantine a primary representation of a particular state of the affairs in the world. You need to cut it off from its direct connection with the outside world. After decoupling it becomes a different kind of representation, which can even be in contradiction to the state of affairs in the world. You can pretend or imagine that something is the case. Leslie has this equation where he says the agent stands in some informational relation (thinks, believes, wishes, pretends) to a state in the world (e.g. it is raining outside). The agent is whatever you make it to be. It could be self, other, a dog or a triangle, as long as you ascribe agency. The famous example is a mother holding up a banana like a telephone and speaking into it. An 18-month-old child can perfectly comprehend this. The child laughs and is not going to be confused about bananas and telephones. Where in the brain might this decoupling be done? We have no idea.

Hauser: I thought you were going to say something stronger than that. Isn't it the case that ontogenetically self-knowledge is coming on line substantially earlier than other-knowledge. There is pretence and appearance reality distinction way before any concept of other minds.

U Frith: Not necessarily. Pretence and the appearance–reality distinction are easier to test at an early age, because we have implicit tests. Concepts of other minds are usually tested with explicit tests and with complex designs. For example, false belief scenarios. Even five-year olds often find these hard to follow.

Hauser: To do the appearance/reality distinction, you need to be able to maintain an alternative perspective. This has nothing to do with other minds. It has to do with you having the capacity to entertain different representational systems independently of other minds.

Gergely: But it doesn't follow from having an early perspective taking ability at another domain that you cannot apply such an ability equally early when thinking about other minds as well.

Hauser: You don't at that age. Appearance/reality comes in before some of the theory-of-mind (ToM) stuff.

Gergely: Now there is evidence of implicit theory of mind in 15-month-olds (Onishi & Baillargeon 2005).

U Frith: The evidence we get depends on finding the right task to tap the competence of the child. I don't know of evidence that would suggest strongly that first of all you would understand your own mental states, and only then would you know something about another person's mental states. The seeing/knowing distinction is a bit like the appearance/reality distinction. When we have done experiments on the seeing/knowing distinction with young children, we have found simultaneously evidence for self and other awareness. For example, if you see a particular object in a closed container, you know what it is, and someone else who has not seen the object, doesn't know. This insight also works in the reverse and can be observed in 3–4 year-olds.

Gallese: What is the age of onset of this capacity?

U Frith: The tasks we commonly use need language, and they can only be done when the child can perform the task. It doesn't mean the child would not already have the competence at an earlier age. When we use looking behaviour instead of verbal responses, we can go down to 3 years, and even, as Baillargeon has shown with an ingenious paradigm, down to 15 months. The capacity to predict the behaviour of a person who has a false belief is apparent already then.

Adolphs: The idea Chris raised that we find out about our own minds based on the capacity of understanding other people's minds seems on the face of it at odds with the idea we heard from Vittorio Gallese that one way we find out about other people is by mapping it on to some kind of a simulation in ourselves. This would assume that we have in place knowledge of what it is that we are doing so we can map other people's actions onto this. There is some kind of tension here.

C Frith: Couldn't you have the following story about how you learn about your emotions. First you see someone making a certain facial expression and being sad, and then you realize that when you make that facial expression you must be sad too.

Adolphs: To recognize that the person is sad, you are mapping it onto some kind of simulation yourself. The prerequisite would seem to be that you know what it is that is going on in yourself in the first place.

Montague: It wouldn't have to be explicit. You could have processors that can mimic without having explicit representation.

Adolphs: It would have to be explicit enough that you can go from what is taking place in yourself to explicit knowledge of what is going on in the other person, since this is the kind of explicit knowledge that we all measure in experiments.

Montague: It wouldn't have to be, you we are talking about having knowledge. It could be automatic.

Adolphs: You are using representations of what is going on in yourself to reconstruct knowledge of what is going on in the other person. It seems to me that the prerequisite for this is that you already have to know what it would be like if you were doing this in the first place to understand what the other person is doing. Or am I missing something here?

Gergely: I don't think this is a conceptual prerequisite. It is a very widely shared intuition, but there are other models. One idea is that contingent emotion mirroring provided by interacting with others, something, by the way, that only humans seem to do, has a kind of social biofeedback function of individuating and building secondary representations for your procedural primary emotional states (Gergely & Watson 1999). Then, eventually, what you have learned about the emotional meaning of facial expressions of others and their dispositional consequences will be possible to use to interpret your own categorical emotions as well. So it is the other way round, just as Chris Frith suggested. You can make a coherent developmental model where it clearly goes the other way round, although this is counterintuitive to most people.

Singer: What about the behavioural data revealing egocentricity bias? You are quicker in detecting writing which is closer to your own writing. When you are thirsty you are quicker in recognizing thirst in other people. I don't know about the ontogeny of how you get your self-representation, but in adult it seems that you use your own representation to understand those of others. That is, you have a bias towards your own experiences.

Gergely: That is another story. The other way round, you are putting in an enormous amount of innate machinery just to understand the other through yourself. Especially if you think in terms of motor competence, it has extremely slow ontogenetic development. So you would be forced to say that you don't understand grasping in other people before you can grasp yourself.

Adolphs: Is that true?

Gergely: No.

Gallese: You shouldn't confound motor competence by confusing the output (what can you tell your muscle to do, which develops later on) with the motor schemata (which are mapped in your brain). If you are congenitally limb deficient you can still experience phantom limb sensations. When these sensations occur, this leads to the activation of the appropriate premotor brain areas.

Gergely: That I accept, but what you couldn't do is understand motor actions that are morphologically different, such as morphed hand movements that you cannot perform or that are, in fact, impossible to perform by humans. There is recent evidence that 6–8 month olds can understand as goal-directed even biologically impossible hand actions. There is also evidence that between 6 and 12 months of age infants understand certain patterns of non-biological movements of even unfamiliar objects (such as a rod) as goal-directed (Király et al 2003).

Gallese: Somerville & Woodward (2005) are showing that infants' motor competence can predict their capacity to understand the intentional structure of observed actions.

C Frith: There is a recent paper by Gunter Knoblich and his colleagues relevant to this (Bosbach et al 2005). They looked at people who were deafferented and thus no longer had any awareness of their own limb movements. These people were still able to recognise when observing an action whether someone was picking up a light or a heavy box. But they were not able to tell whether the person picking up the box had been misled about the weight of the box. In this case the box lifter has to make unanticipated postural adjustments which can be detected by normal observers. I have no idea what this means but it seems deeply relevant.

Call: The self knowledge/other knowledge distinction is an interesting one because most work has been done on other knowledge: attributing mental states or attribution to others. Very little has been done on self knowledge. There is room for having some access to self-knowledge. For example, it would be of interest to an organism to have access to whether they have forgotten the place where certain foods are. There are now data showing that primates can do both the self and other, and other species like pigeons and dogs can do the other but they can't do the self.

Macrae: What is the test? Is it the mirror test?

Call: No, it's not the mirror test. It is about perspective taking. They can take the perspective of others, but then when they are put in a situation where they have to assess what they have seen themselves, they don't take that information into account.

Macrae: It strikes me that there is a huge experimental mismatch. There is a growing industry of ever-cleverer ways of working out what is going on in another person's mind, getting earlier and earlier in the developmental trajectory. This isn't seen in the self literature, however. This mismatch makes it difficult to draw any definitive conclusions.

C Frith: Is that a technical problem?

Macrae: Yes. Perhaps one day someone in this room will have a killer paradigm for self-knowledge that will change the weight that we are giving to these respective findings.

De Vignemont: The simulation theory assumes most of the time a priority of the self for understanding the others. However, Robert Gordon (1996) defends a different version of the simulation theory, what he calls the 'ascent routine'. According to him, you don't need to look inwardly at your own mental states, all you need is to look outwardly at the external world. If I want to know whether I believe that it is raining, I don't need to introspect, I just look out the window. The problem with this strategy is that it works only for beliefs: rather than to ask 'do you believe *p*?', you ask 'is *p* true?'. But it doesn't work for desire, for instance because there is no question equivalent, which would not appeal to the mental concept of desire. The only way to know your own desire is to look inwardly. In addition, when you have competitive desires, you need to know which one has priority if you want to act accordingly. For example, a child might desire both a carrot cake and a chocolate cake, and he cannot decide which one he wants just by looking to the others or to the cakes.

Macrae: There was a long tradition in self perception theory that suggested that the only basis we have to understand ourselves is to look at our behaviour in context and look to others for cues about what we think and feel. In some contexts this seems reasonable, but in others it is questionable whether self-knowledge is gleaned in this manner.

C Frith: One of the next steps in the work you were talking about is to ask the question as to whether there are distinctions between different kinds of mental states, such as beliefs and desires. This could be in terms of the systems involved. To what extent do the kinds of studies you described look at those distinctions? Are all these different mental states lumped together?

Macrae: There is an interesting question. For the last 15 years in social-cognition research, automaticity has been the hot topic. Some people have suggested that everything that is interesting in the domain of person perception is the product of some unconditionally automatic mental operation. There are lines of behavioural evidence that supply some support for this viewpoint. However, if you think about the ensuing cognitive chaos that would arise if the social mind operated in this manner, there needs to be some regulatory mechanism in place to keep social cognition from spinning out of control. In some domains of social cognition, for example person categorisation and stereotyping, researchers have now identified those mechanisms. The same may be true of this notion of whether we spontaneously automatically mentalize when we interact with others. If we don't, what are the contexts or conditions under which we don't? This turns out to be an important issue. If we don't mentalize, then we could deny that people are moral beings. There is a broad issue therefore about the boundary conditions for when we do and don't mentalize about others.

Montague: What do you mean by 'automatic'?

Macrae: The classic view in social cognition is that many social-cognitive effects are stimulus driven: a stimulus falls on your retina, then various cognitive processes will get to work in an obligatory and unstoppable way.

Montague: If you had an executive process that is modulated by a lot of variables, and itself could control a lot of processes, but you could capture it in a set of equations, is that automatic? It seems to me that everything for which you could have a quantitative description becomes functionally describable as automatic.

Macrae: Let me give an example. The instant that you perceive me, you would automatically and inevitably have access to any information you have in your memory about Scottish people. In social cognition this has been one of the classic definitions of an automatic social-cognitive event.

Montague: At some point we will have quantitative descriptions of these many levels. Lots of the magic will be chased into an ever-smaller corner.

C Frith: Some people try to capture the nature of automaticity by contrasting bottom-up processes with top-down processes. Bottom-up processes are more automatic. The more you can modulate a process by context the less automatic it is in some sense. This depends, of course, on what you mean by context. In the sort of work that Neil Macrae is describing, they are now asking whether there are top–down mechanisms in the brain which modulate how much emotion you have.

Macrae: I think the real contribution that social cognition research can make to this debate is in the introduction of top–down forces. Everyday social life is inherently top–down. It's not to say that a bottom–up argument isn't going to take you far, rather that the last mile will be hugely interesting and that is where top–down modulatory forces become interesting.

Gallese: Your paper was interesting because it puts many controversial issues on the table. I suspect that mentalizing (both trying to find out what other people think and what is self-centred) is a multilayered process. If we look for the neural correlate of mentalizing as such we may end up with the controversial results we are facing now. There are different degrees we may enter when we are facing the behaviour of others. Most of the time we are following predictions. As long as these predictions are fulfilled it is a smooth process that doesn't require the investment of huge cognitive resources. But when something doesn't fit with the prediction, we may introduce new cognitive processes which may be mapped in different parts of the brain. The same applies to our phenomenal awareness. People looking at this have distinguished levels. A common experience I have is that my facial mimicry doesn't match with my inner mood feeling. Sometimes, I am asked by people, 'why are you angry with me?' when I am not. This tells us that the level of our knowledge of our own state isn't sure. This relies most likely on the activation of different brain circuitries.

Macrae: I would agree. The other frustrating thing from a social cognition perspective is that you come to appreciate that the kinds of processes involved are hugely underspecified. We simply don't know what the component processes may be.

Gergely: In developmental psychopathology there are a number of affective self-disorders where there is a severe deficit in understanding ones own emotional states. They don't necessarily involve a corresponding deficit in understanding others.

Hauser: I see the comment you made about how these things work on other minds to the neglect of self as being truely independent of the imaging data. How does this contribute to a coming together of that information that couldn't be had by pure developmental data or psychopathological data? What does the brain piece add to this particular part of the story?

Macrae: Apart from colour pictures and an easy way to spend lots of money? For us, this is a dependent measure that is really usefully applied to some questions in this domain in a search for converging evidence, but for other questions it is hopeless. Part of the struggle some people are having with social cognitive neuroscience is that it is frequently applied in spectacular but essentially non-theoretical domains. It is a struggle to get tractable empirical problems where fMRI can be useful. Where it has been particularly useful is in the self domain. In this area there has been a lively debate about whether there is anything special or different about self, or are enhanced memory effects in the self domain just driven by classic levels of processing effects. Now we have imaging evidence to suggest that it is not simply a matter of levels of processing, self-referential processing has some interesting neural properties.

Hauser: When you did the animated versus the real version, is the difference one of attention? Is the attention mediating the difference, or is it something about the nature of the representation?

Macrae: There are some suggestions that people may engage in imagery-based processing when thinking about animated agents, but ToM processing when thinking about real people.

Hauser: This is where some of the developmental psychology literature has done terrifically well in teasing apart what triggers different attributions about agencies. This is getting at the primitives that launch the response.

Frank: Does the understanding of autism shed any light on the priority of development of self versus others? Autistic children don't have a very good ToM, but presumably know what they want. Is there the contrary malady: an individual who has a good theory of what other people want but not of their own wants?

Macrae: Has anyone done the classic self-referencing paradigm on autistic individuals? If so, do they show the self-reference effect in memory? This is if you are given a bunch of items to rate, and if you rate the items in the context of a hypothetical other, generally there is an enhancement for items previously rated in a self-referential manner. This is pretty robust effect.

U Frith: That is a great idea. No one has done it.

Macrae: This speaks to the relationship of notions of self in some of these populations that are believed to be hugely influential in shaping our understanding of person perception. But what about the process of self perception in these individuals?

Van Lange: In a lot of paradigms the other is salient, so this draws attention to the other. But if you have a paradigm where you ask about preferences, a stable finding is that people use themselves to get that judgment about others. For example, if you ask undergraduates how many people eat Chinese food once a week they will overestimate it because they eat Chinese more often than other people, in the Netherlands at least. People use the self as an anchor for reaching judgments about others.

Moll: I'd like to come back to a point I mentioned yesterday; for me, it *does* make sense that you use the same knowledge for self and others. It wouldn't be interesting for the brain to have double, or multiple representations of exactly the same type of knowledge, used for both self and others. If the brain stores features or semantic knowledge of persons and events, wouldn't it be interesting to retrieve this knowledge from the same locations where it is stored?

Macrae: No, it is not so much the level of representations, but rather the process level. Clearly, semantic memory and autobiographical memory are different beasts. It is the level of component processes you bring to bear when you seek to understand social objects in your world, whether they be self or other people. What are these component processes, and to what extent are they shared across different classes of stimuli?

Gallese: I have a possible answer to your question. This lies in what Daniel Stern has called 'vitality affect'. This is the dynamic temporal profile of the stimulus that from the early stages of our cognitive development we can cross-modally map on our body. Be it a tactile stimulus with a peculiar roughness, or presented in a visual modality, there are temporal contours that our brain is wired up to recognize and pin down. One interesting experiment would be to find a neural correlate of this temporal profile regardless of the stimulus. This is something I am thinking about.

Macrae: One way of getting at this would be to ask to what extent does perceived similarity to targets matter? There could be a kinship hypothesis: if people look a little bit like you, you are more likely to employ some ToM strategies than others. One of the things we are doing is using morphing to create targets that resemble self to varying degrees. Then when you encounter these targets, how important is the similarity overlap? This begins to probe at the edges of these sorts of issues.

Gergely: I have a point about autism. One piece of evidence that many believe is relevant in this regard is that children with autism pass the mirror self recognition test (i.e. when they notice in the mirror a red rouge spot on their face that had inadvertently been placed there before without their knowledge, they try to rub it off from their actual face rather than from the face in the mirror). Many have interpreted this as evidence that they have a concept of self. However, this capacity doesn't correlate with understanding other minds as shown by their severe deficit in mind-reading. However, there are a number of alternative explanations for passing the mirror self recognition test that doesn't involve having a self concept (see Gergely 1994). So I don't think this is the right interpretation that they have of self. The other relevant piece of evidence is that autistic individuals are not sensitive to their names in the same way as normal children. By four and a half months human infants react to their own names. This sensitivity is highly impaired in autistic children.

Sigman: It is amazing to see autistic children who have so little ability in self recognition, yet they recognize a distortion in their body image instantly.

U Frith: We have been thinking about this apparent puzzle in autism in relation to their clearly egocentric stance. Frederique De Vignemont has some ideas on how to resolve this puzzle.

De Vignemont: The hypothesis that we defend with Uta Frith concerns individuals with Asperger syndrome (cf. Frith & de Vignemont 2005). They are able to pass the false-belief task and yet, they have clear difficulties in social interaction. How can we account for that? We apply to social cognition the spatial distinction between egocentric and allocentric representations. We suggest that there are two ways to understand people. On the one hand, I can understand someone I am interacting with. On the other hand, I can understand the same person when she is in interaction with someone else. In the former case, one adopts an egocentric stance where the other is understood relative to the self. In the latter case, one adopts an allocentric stance because one represents a relationship between two agents independently of the self. We think that these two stances are disconnected in people with Asperger syndrome, whereas in most people they are in constant interaction. People with Asperger take an extreme egocentric stance and their social life is self-centred. At the same time, because of this disconnection, they have an extreme allocentrism and their understanding of other people is completely detached and unrelated to their past interaction with them. This leads to a disturbed view of how the social world works.

Macrae: That is interesting. Translating that line of argument into self-referencing and memory produces spectacular predictions about how these individuals might perform.

Call: Do children with autism know when they have forgotten something?

U Frith: You are referring to Tulving's autonoetic memory. This type of memory has been investigated rather rarely. You would expect it to be impaired if this type of awareness of your own ability to remember something was related to ToM.

C Frith: Are you thinking about the experiments with monkeys by Hampton (2001), where, if the monkey got the opportunity to indicate that they couldn't remember the answer, they could actually do better, because they could eliminate wrong guesses. I don't think this has ever been done in autism.

I have a brain imaging question. In your experiments with the cartoon versus the real films, there is a general and interesting problem about how you interpret changes in activity. If you present people with words, then the visual word form area lights up. If you present people with non-words based on real words then this area activates even more. The argument would be that this is because it is working harder to try to discover what the stimuli are. When you do your real film versus your cartoon film, you could argue that there should be areas that have to work harder to understand what is going on in the cartoon because it is in some sense degraded. How do you decide which is the important area to look at: the one where activity goes up or the one activity goes down?

Macrae: One of my collaborators was wedded to the view that when he watches any form of cartoon his brain is working harder as he tries to understand what is going on. His belief was that if you did the cartoon greater than real contrast you would see more activity in the theory of mind network. We didn't observe this. Instead we saw activity in areas associated with visual processing. Again this relates to the general question of whether we mentalize for all types of stimuli or only specific targets? Right now, this is an open question.

Montague: Your imaging would be averaging over all these possibilities, and showing us the bulk difference.

Moll: I wonder whether there is a baseline issue with your imaging data. I would expect that you would find strong activation in more dorsal occiptotemporal areas for the cartoons, including in the superior temporal sulcus regions, if not arising from theory-of-mind-related mechanisms, but at least from the presence of biological movement.

Macrae: We matched clips as closely as possible.

Adolphs: Did you do quantitative measures on how well all these stimuli were matched, such as the motion cues or luminance?

Macrae: Yes. It took 6 months to create the movie segments. But there may be subtle stimulus properties that are different across the two versions of the movie.

Montague: What was you claim for the inferior frontal gyrus (IFG)?

Macrae: In my amateur understanding of mirror neurons, I worry about a system that fires off all the time. Surely it would have me preparing for irrelevant action in many circumstances. If there were a braking system that could say 'hold on, you are resonating to the world but in a situation that is not really optimal', this would be useful. Perhaps activity in IFG is performing such an inhibitory act.

Blakemore: What was your interpretation of the superior temporal sulcus (STS) and the temporal parietal junction (TPJ) activity?

Macrae: I am not sure that I necessarily agree with Rebecca Saxe's take on the role of the TPJ in mentalizing, although her argument is interesting. As for STS, it is modulated by biological motion but more so for real than animated agents in our study. TPJ is found in all sorts of ToM imaging experiments, but I am just not sure what the functional story is for activity in that region. There are at least two groups that have different views; I'm agnostic.

Sigman: In terms of autism, Uta Frith and I have parallel findings at different ages. There was a time when I visited her and told her about our findings, and she told me about hers. They found this problem with ToM and about the same time we found this problem in joint attention. I always thought that we would be able to see continuity, because we would see the same children, follow them until they were older, and then measure their ToM. We would find continuing difficulties. This didn't work out in practice because too few of our children developed enough language ability to do the ToM tasks, so we couldn't look at this. What seems to be happening in the brain imaging literature is that we are finding the same areas of deficit when we look at ToM and joint attention. These two processes may be linked.

Macrae: For many social cognition folks the 'where' question is much less interesting than the 'when' question. People are trying to discern which of these social-cognitive strategies are coming on really fast. This may help unlock many of these mysteries. We are now slowly trying to design experiments that will exploit this sort of technology to get at the temporal story as well.

C Frith: There is a brain imaging experiment on joint attention from David Perrett's group (Williams et al 2005). It is not quite joint attention but it is as close as you can get in an fMRI scanner. The subjects have to follow a target with their eyes and they see someone else who is either following the same target with their eyes or not. It seems to light up much the same system as ToM tasks.

Montague: Have these ToM tasks been done in parallel on a box or computer? Say I watch a computer output or I have a box that generates something, have people done imaging experiments with this? How fast do you assign a 'mind' to something that doesn't have one? For example, I was watching a hornets nest, and this follows a series of rules (when they fly in or out, when they are aggressive or not, what they'll do if I touch it), so there's a sense that it has internal 'mental' structure. I have machinery in my head that lets me make inferences about this. Surely this is related to the machinery I use to decide what it is in people's heads. Have people done these mentalizing tasks in scanners?

Adolphs: There have indeed been experiments using abstract animations that seem to engage mentalizing mechanisms. They do engage mentalizing for things that aren't people. Presumably the explanation of the findings is that you make lots of complex predictions about things in the world, and the real question is whether there is a kind of threshold that is reached which taps into this mentalizing system that has evolved for predicting the behaviour of other people. How far do we have to go in the features of the stimuli before this kicks in?

U Frith: In all of these tasks the really interesting conditions are the controls. We have animations that do not trigger your attributional systems.

Adolphs: That's right: there are some cues that trigger and some that don't.

Montague: I guess the threshold is the interesting issue.

Adolphs: And it is interesting from two points of view. First, it is interesting to know what it is about the stimuli (what kind of biological motion cues are needed and so on) and second it is interesting to know what it is from the point of view of the perceiver: there will be individual differences in the propensity with which you make the attributions.

Montague: No one has done an experiment where this has been paramaterized and the threshold identified.

Hauser: It has psychophysically. Brian Scholl's (Scholl 2001, Scholl & Tremoulet 2000) work has begun to titrate dimensions along which you do or do not see an object as an object.

References

Bosbach S, Cole J, Prinz W, Knoblich G 2005 Inferring another's expectation from action: the role of peripheral sensation. Nat Neurosci 8:1295–1297

Frith U, de Vignemont F 2005 Egocentrism, Allocentrism and Asperger syndrome. Consciousness Cognit 14:719–738

Gergely G 1994 From self-recognition to theory of mind. In: Parker S, Mitchell R, Boccia M (eds) Self-Awareness in animals and humans: developmental perspectives. Cambridge University Press, p 51–61

Gergely G, Watson JS 1999 Early social-emotional development: Contingency perception and the social biofeedback model. In: Rochat P (ed) Early social cognition. Erlbaum, Hillsdale NJ, p 101–137

Gordon RM 1996 Simulation without introspection or inference from me to you. In: Carruthers P, Smith P (eds) Theories of theories of mind. Cambridge University Press, Cambridge

Hampton RR 2001 Rhesus monkeys know when they remember. Proc Natl Acad Sci USA 98:5359–5362

Happe F 2003 Theory of mind and the self. Ann N Y Acad Sci 1001:134–144

Király I, Jovanovic B, Aschersleben G, Prinz W, Gergely G 2003 Generality and perceptual constraints in understanding goal-directed actions in young infants. Consciousness Cognit 12:752–769

Onishi KH, Baillargeon R 2005 Do 15-month-old infants understand false beliefs? Science 308:255–258

Scholl BJ 2001 Objects and attention: The state of the art. Cognition 80:1–46

Scholl BJ, Tremoulet PD 2000 Perceptual causality and animacy. Trends Cog Sci 4:299–309

Sommerville JA, Woodward AL 2005 Pulling out the intentional structure of action: the relation between action processing and action production in infancy. Cognition 95:1–30

Williams JH, Waiter GD, Perra O, Perrett DI, Whiten A 2005 An fMRI study of joint attention experience. Neuroimage 25:133–140

Dissociable systems for empathy

R. J. R. Blair

Mood and Anxiety Disorders Program, National Institute of Mental Health, National Institutes of Heath, Department of Health and Human Services, 15K North Drive, Room 206, MSC 2670, Bethesda, MD 20892–2670, USA

Abstract. Empathy is a lay term that is becoming increasingly used in the field of cognitive neuroscience. In this paper, it is argued that empathy is a loose collection of partially dissociable neurocognitive systems. Two forms of 'emotional' empathy were considered: First, responding to emotional expressions, particularly angry expressions, leading to response reversal. Secondly, responding to emotional expressions, particularly fearful and sad expressions, leading to stimulus–reinforcement learning. The implications of these forms of empathy for understanding specific psychiatric conditions are briefly considered.

2006 Empathy and Fairness. Wiley, Chichester (Novartis Foundation Symposium 278) p 134–145

To some, empathy is considered to be a unitary process. For example, Preston & de Waal (2002) have argued that 'empathy [is] a super-ordinate category that includes all sub-classes of phenomena that share the same mechanism. This includes emotional contagion, sympathy, cognitive empathy, helping behaviour, etc.' (Preston & de Waal 2002 p 4). However, that position will not be supported here. Elsewhere (Blair 2005), I have argued that the term 'empathy' subsumes a variety of dissociable neurocognitive processes. I have previously considered three main divisions, each reliant on at least partially dissociable neural systems: cognitive, motor and emotional empathy (Blair 2005). The goal of the current paper is narrower. In this paper, two forms of emotional empathy will be considered: (1) responses to emotional expressions, particularly angry expressions, leading to response reversal; and (2) responses to emotional expressions, particularly fearful and sad expressions, leading to stimulus–reinforcement learning.

The current paper makes one fundamental assumption: facial expressions of emotion have a communicatory function and that they impart specific information to the observer (see also, Blair 2003, see also, 2005, Fridlund 1991). This does not imply that the display of an emotional expression implies an intention in the expresser to convey a specific message to the observer. Instead, the argument is simply that emotional expressions convey information on the valence of objects/situations between conspecifics rapidly. Thus, important triggers for an emotional display include both an emotional event and also a potential observer. If there is no observer, the emotional display will either not occur or be considerably muted (see Fridlund 1991).

The literature on social referencing particularly illustrates the communicatory function of emotional expressions (Klinnert et al 1987, Walker-Andrews 1998). When an infant, from the age of eight to 10 months, encounters a novel object, he/she will look towards the primary caregiver and their behaviour will be determined by the caregiver's emotional display. If the caregiver displays an expression of fear or disgust, the child will avoid the novel object. If the caregiver displays a happy expression, the child will approach the novel object. Social referencing is also seen in chimpanzees (Russell et al 1997) and a very similar process has been shown in other monkeys and labelled observational fear (Mineka & Cook 1993). From the above view, emotional empathy to facial and vocal emotional expressions is the 'translation' of the communication by the observer. It is argued that because of the different implications of these communicatory signals they are translated in several separable neurocognitive systems (Blair 2003). Two of these will be considered below.

Social response reversal and the reaction to the anger of others

I have referred to the first of these systems for the 'translation of' and response to specific emotional expressions as the system for social response reversal (SRR); (Blair 2003, Blair & Cipolotti 2000). This system is considered to be activated by aversive social cues (particularly, but not limited to, angry expressions) or expectations of such cues (as would be engendered by representations previously associated with such cues; i.e. representations of actions that make other individuals' angry). This system is considered to (1) guide the individual away from committing conventional transgressions (particularly in the presence of higher status individuals); and (2) orchestrate a response to witnessed conventional transgressions (particularly when these are committed by lower status individuals) (Blair & Cipolotti 2000).

The idea is that the SRR evolved as a system for the resolution of hierarchy interactions between conspecifics. In line with the position, it has been suggested that the human angry expression evolved to mimic a high status dominant face (Marsh et al 2005). Within species aggression in most mammalian species is mediated by subcortical structures also involved in the basic response to threat (Gregg & Siegel 2001, Panksepp 1998). The suggestion is that the SRR is involved in the modulation of this aggressive response; increasing its probability under certain circumstances or decreasing its probability under others.

The activity of the SRR system is thought to be modulated by information on hierarchy and mental state (the latter provided by systems involved in theory of mind [ToM]) (Berthoz et al 2002, Blair & Cipolotti 2000). The form of modulation will be dependent on whether the individual is the perpetrator of (or considering being the perpetrator of), or is the witness to, the conventional transgression (Blair et al 2006).

This work on emotional modulation of appropriate social behaviour has interesting potential links with work on the social emotion of embarrassment. Leary (Leary et al 1996) and others (Gilbert 1997, Keltner & Anderson 2000) have suggested that embarrassment serves an important social function by signalling appeasement to others. When a person's untoward behaviour threatens his/her standing in an important social group, visible signs of embarrassment function as a non-verbal acknowledgement of shared social standards. Leary and Keltner argue that embarrassment displays diffuse negative social evaluations and the likelihood of retaliation and there is a good deal of empirical evidence to support this 'appeasement' or remedial function of embarrassment from studies of both humans and non-human primates (for reviews, see (Gilbert 1997, Keltner & Anderson 2000, Leary et al 1996).

A major neural system thought to be implicated in SRR is ventrolateral prefrontal cortex (Brodmann's Area 47); (Blair & Cipolotti 2000, Blair et al 1999). The suggestion is that this region responds to aversive social cues or expectations of such cues and augments the activity of motor responses alternative to the response currently initiated/about to be initiated (cf. Luo et al 2006). This region is particularly responsive to: (1) angry expressions, as well as other emotional expressions (Blair et al 1999, Sprengelmeyer et al 1998); (2) the individual's own anger (Dougherty et al 1999); (3) consideration of embarrassing situations (Takahashi et al 2004); and (4) transgressions that are likely to result in the anger of others (i.e. conventional transgressions or 'fairness' violations) (Berthoz et al 2002, Fiddick et al 2005). Patients with damage to this region show difficulties with (1) expression recognition (Blair & Cipolotti 2000, Hornak et al 2003, 1996); (2) increased levels of anger (Grafman et al 1996); (3) responding to the embarrassment of others (Beer et al 2003); and (4) when evaluating transgressions that elicit anger in observers (Blair & Cipolotti 2000, Stone et al 2002).

I have argued that disruption in the functioning of the SRR underpins many of the phenomena associated with what Damasio (1994) termed acquired sociopathy; i.e. the increase in frustration/threat based aggression and inappropriate social behaviour (Blair 2004). Damasio (1994) has suggested that acquired sociopathy might be considered an acquired form of developmental psychopathy. Individuals with psychopathy are marked by pronounced emotional (considerably reduced empathy and guilt) and behavioural disturbance (criminal activity and, frequently, violence); (Hare 1991). Psychopathy is a developmental disorder in that it usually appears in early childhood (certainly by eight years of age) and continues throughout the lifespan (Harpur & Hare 1994).

Psychopathy has long been considered a disorder of empathy (Hare 1991). However, I will argue not of the form of empathy described by the SRR model. There are marked differences between the functional impairments associated with, and the behavioral presentation of, acquired sociopathy and developmental psychopathy (see Blair 2004). However, in contrast, there appear to be marked similarities between the functional impairments associated with, and the behavioural presentation of, acquired sociopathy and childhood bipolar disorder (see Blair 2005).

Responding to the fear and sadness of others and the emergence of care based morality

The second system for the 'translation of' and response to specific emotional expressions involves the amygdala and is considered crucial for the development of care-based morality. I have argued that two functional processes are necessary for the emergence of care based morality: First, an intact 'empathic response' to the fear and distress of others and; Secondly, the ability of form stimulus-reinforcement associations. Without an aversive response to victim's distress, the individual will not learn actions that are associated with victims' distress are bad. Moreover, the individual will only learn that actions associated with victim's distress are bad, if they can perform stimulus (representation of action)–reinforcement (victim's distress) associations. Both of these processes rely on the functional integrity of the amygdala. I argue that disruption to these processes, as a result of the amygdala dysfunction, leads to the development of psychopathy (Blair 2004).

Considerable neuroimaging and neuropsychological work shows the role of the amygdala in responding to fearful and, to a lesser extent, sad expressions (Adolphs 2002, Blair et al 1999, Drevets et al 2000). Moreover, considerable human and animal neuroimaging and neuropsychological work shows the role of the amygdala in stimulus–reinforcement learning (Baxter & Murray 2002, Kosson et al 2006, O'Doherty et al 2002). Individuals with psychopathy show impairment in the recognition of fearful and to a lesser extent sad expressions (Blair et al 2001) and reduced amygdala responses to such expressions (Gordon et al 2004). Moreover, individuals with psychopathy show impairment in stimulus–reinforcement learning (Newman & Kosson 1986) and reduced amygdala responses during such learning (Birbaumer et al 2005).

In short, the argument is that the amygdala allows individuals to learn that specific actions/objects are either good or bad to conduct according to whether these actions/objects are associated with either the recipient's happiness or the victim's distress. Following Schoenbaum and colleagues (Gallagher et al 1999, Pickens et al 2003), the suggestion is made that the amygdala passes information on the expected reinforcement associated with a particular object/action (aversion induced by a potential victim's distress or reward induced by observed happiness) to medial orbital frontal cortex (Blair 2004, Kosson et al 2006). Using this information, medial orbital frontal cortex initiates approach to, or withdrawal from, the object/action.

The argument then is that once the individual has learnt about a prosocial behaviour/transgression, representation of the action will elicit an integrated emotional response that includes both the amygdala and medial orbital frontal cortex. This emotional response is effectively the individual's automatic 'moral attitude' to the representation (c.f. Luo et al 2006). In line with this position, recent neuroimaging studies of morality using different methodologies such as an morality Implicit Association Test (Luo et al 2006), making moral decisions based on text descriptions of ethical dilemmas (Greene et al 2004, 2001), passive viewing pictures of moral violations (Moll et al 2002b), judging sentence descriptions of behaviours as moral or immoral (Heekeren et al 2005, Moll et al 2002a) and making moral decisions (morally appropriate or not) versus semantic decisions (semantically correct or not) on sentences (Heekeren et al 2003) have implicated both the amygdala and medial regions of orbital frontal cortex.

Conclusions

Empathy is a lay term that has been used to describe many different neurocognitive functions. Three broad categories can be distinguished: ToM, motor empathy and emotional empathy (Blair 2005). Within this paper, two forms of emotional empathy were considered: First, responses to emotional expressions, particularly angry expressions, leading to response reversal. Disruption in this form of 'empathic' reaction is considered to lead to problems in (a) modulating behaviour as a consequence of other individuals' social cues; (b) anger regulation; (c) responding to other individuals' embarrassment and feeling embarrassment in the self; and (d) evaluating transgressions that elicit anger in observers and modulating behaviour accordingly. I argued that individuals with acquired sociopathy have problems with this type of empathic response. I also argued that a developmental pathology linked to disruption in this form of empathic response is childhood bipolar disorder.

The second form of emotional empathy involved responding to emotional expressions, particularly fearful and sad expressions, leading to stimulus–reinforcement learning. I argued that disruption in the systems necessary for this form of 'empathic' reaction lead to problems in (a) responding to the fearful and sad expressions of others; and (b) stimulus–reinforcement learning. I also argued that a developmental pathology linked to disruption in this form of empathic response is developmental psychopathy.

In short, empathy is a general term for a collection of specific neurocognitive functions that can be disrupted selectively and which, when disrupted, can lead to specific psychiatric disorders, such as childhood bipolar disorder and psychopathy. By understanding empathy, we are likely to be able to understand, and therefore treat, these disorders.

Acknowledgements

This research was supported by the Intramural Research Program of the NIH: NIMH

References

Adolphs R 2002 Neural systems for recognizing emotion. Curr Opin Neurobiol 12:169–177

Baxter MG, Murray EA 2002 The amygdala and reward. Nat Rev Neurosci 3:563–573

Beer JS, Heeray EA, Keltner D, Scabini D, Knight RT 2003 The regulatory function of self-conscious emotion: Insights from patients with orbitofrontal damage. J Pers Soc Psychol 85:594–604

Berthoz S, Armony J, Blair RJR, Dolan R 2002 Neural correlates of violation of social norms and embarrassment. Brain 125:1696–1708

Birbaumer N, Veit R, Lotze M et al 2005 Deficient fear conditioning in psychopathy: A functional magnetic resonance imaging study. Arch Gen Psychiatry 62:799–805

Blair RJR 2003 Facial expressions, their communicatory functions and neuro-cognitive substrates. Philos Trans R Soc Lond B Biol Sci 358:561–572

Blair RJR 2004 The roles of orbital frontal cortex in the modulation of antisocial behavior. Brain Cogn 55:198–208

Blair RJ 2005 Responding to the emotions of others: dissociating forms of empathy through the study of typical and atypical populations. Conscious Cogn 14:698–718

Blair RJR, Cipolotti L 2000 Impaired social response reversal: A case of 'acquired sociopathy'. Brain 123:1122–1141

Blair RJR, Morris JS, Frith CD, Perrett DI, Dolan R 1999 Dissociable neural responses to facial expressions of sadness and anger. Brain 122:883–893

Blair RJR, Colledge E, Murray L, Mitchell DG 2001 A selective impairment in the processing of sad and fearful expressions in children with psychopathic tendencies. J Abnorm Child Psychol 29:491–498

Blair RJR, Marsh AA, Finger E, Blair KS, Luo Q 2006 Neuro-cognitive systems involved in morality. Philosophical Explorations 9:13–27

Damasio AR 1994 Descartes' error: Emotion, rationality and the human brain. Putnam (Grosset Books), New York

Dougherty DD, Shin LM, Alpert NM et al 1999 Anger in healthy men: a PET study using script-driven imagery. Biol Psychiatry 1999 46:466–472

Drevets WC, Lowry T, Gautier C, Perrett DI, Kupfer DJ 2000 Amygdalar blood flow responses to facially expressed sadness. Biol Psychiatry 47:160S

Fiddick L, Spampinato MV, Grafman J 2005 Social contracts and precautions activate different neurological systems: An FMRI investigation of deontic reasoning. Neuroimage 28:778–786

Fridlund AJ 1991 Sociality of solitary smiling: Potentiation by an implicit audience. J Pers Soc Psychol 60:229–246

Gallagher M, McMahan RW, Schoenbaum G 1999 Orbitofrontal cortex and representation of incentive value in associative learning. J Neurosci 19:6610–6614

Gilbert P 1997 The evolution of social attractiveness and its role in shame, humiliation, guilt and therapy. Br J Med Psychol 70:113–147

Gordon HL, Baird AA, End A 2004 Functional differences among those high and low on a trait measure of psychopathy. Biol Psychiatry 56:516–521

Grafman J, Schwab K, Warden D, Pridgen BS, Brown HR 1996 Frontal lobe injuries, violence, and aggression: A report of the Vietnam head injury study. Neurology 46:1231–1238

Greene JD, Sommerville RB, Nystrom LE, Darley JM, Cohen JD 2001 An fMRI investigation of emotional engagement in moral judgment. Science 293:1971–1972

Greene JD, Nystrom LE, Engell AD, Darley JM, Cohen JD 2004 The neural bases of cognitive conflict and control in moral judgment. Neuron 44:389–400

Gregg TR, Siegel A 2001 Brain structures and neurotransmitters regulating aggression in cats: implications for human aggression. Prog Neuropsychopharmacol Biol Psychiatry 25: 91–140

Hare RD 1991 The hare psychopathy checklist-revised. Multi-health systems. Toronto, Ontario

Harpur TJ, Hare RD 1994 Assessment of psychopathy as a function of age. J Abnorm Psychol 103:604–609

Heekeren HR, Wartenburger I, Schmidt H, Schwintowski HP, Villringer A 2003 An fMRI study of simple ethical decision-making. Neuroreport 14:1215–1219

Heekeren HR, Wartenburger I, Schmidt H, Prehn K, Schwintowski HP, Villringer A 2005 Influence of bodily harm on neural correlates of semantic and moral decision-making. Neuroimage 24:887–897

Hornak J, Rolls ET, Wade D 1996 Face and voice expression identification in patients with emotional and behavioural changes following ventral frontal damage. Neuropsychologia 34: 247–261

Hornak J, Bramham J, Rolls ET et al 2003 Changes in emotion after circumscribed surgical lesions of the orbitofrontal and cingulate cortices. Brain 126:1691–1712

Keltner D, Anderson C 2000 Saving face for Darwin: The functions and uses of embarrassment. Current Directions in Psychological Science 9:187–192

Klinnert MD, Emde RN, Butterfield P, Campos JJ 1987 Social referencing: The infant's use of emotional signals from a friendly adult with mother present. Annual Progress in Child Psychiatry and Child Development 22:427–432

Kosson DS, Budhani S, Nakic M et al 2006 The role of the amygdala and rostral anterior cingulate in encoding expected outcomes during learning. Neuroimage 29:1161–1172

Leary MR, Landel JL, Patton KM 1996 The motivated expression of embarrassment following a self-presentational predicament. J Pers 64:619–637

Luo Q, Nakic M, Wheatley T, Richell R, Martin A, Blair RJR 2006 The neural basis of implicit moral attitude - an IAT study using event-related fMRI. Neuroimage 30:1449–1457

Marsh AA, Adams RB, Kleck RE 2005 Why do fear and anger look the way they do? From and social function in facial expressions. Pers Soc Psychol Bull 31:1–14

Mineka S, Cook M 1993 Mechanisms involved in the observational conditioning of fear. J Exp Psychol Gen 122:23–38

Moll J, De Oliveira-Souza R, Bramati IE, Grafman J 2002a Functional networks in emotional moral and nonmoral social judgments. Neuroimage 16:696–703

Moll J, de Oliveira-Souza R, Eslinger PJ et al 2002b The neural correlates of moral sensitivity: a functional magnetic resonance imaging investigation of basic and moral emotions. J Neurosci 22:2730–2736

Newman JP, Kosson DS 1986 Passive avoidance learning in psychopathic and nonpsychopathic offenders. J Abnorm Psychol 95:252–256

O'Doherty JP, Deichmann R, Critchley HD, Dolan RJ 2002 Neural responses during anticipation of a primary taste reward. Neuron 33:815–826

Panksepp J 1998 Affective neuroscience: The foundations of human and animal emotions. Oxford University Press, New York

Pickens CL, Saddoris MP, Setlow B, Gallagher M, Holland PC, Schoenbaum G 2003 Different roles for orbitofrontal cortex and basolateral amygdala in a reinforcer devaluation task. J Neurosci 23:11078–11094

Preston SD, de Waal FB 2002 Empathy: Its ultimate and proximate bases. Behav Brain Sci Behav 25:1–20

Russell CL, Bard KA, Adamson LB 1997 Social referencing by young chimpanzees (Pan troglodytes). J Comp Psychol 111:185–193

Sprengelmeyer R, Rausch M, Eysel UT, Przuntek H 1998 Neural structures associated with the recognition of facial basic emotions. Proc R Soc Lond B Biol Sci 265:1927–1931

Stone VE, Cosmides L, Tooby J, Kroll N, Knight RT 2002 Selective impairment of reasoning about social exchange in a patient with bilateral limbic system damage. Proc Natl Acad Sci USA 99:11531–11536

Takahashi HH, Yahata NN, Koeda MM, Matsuda TT, Asai KK, Okubo YY 2004 Brain activation associated with evaluative processes of guilt and embarrassment: an fMRI study. NeuroImage 23:967

Walker-Andrews AS 1998 Emotions and social development: Infants' recognition of emotions in others. Pediatrics 102:1268–1271

DISCUSSION

C Frith: Where does the problem come from?

Blair: There are several studies all showing a strong heritability for the emotional problems. There used to be a long literature on the genetics of violence and antisocial behaviour. This culminated with the most bizarre bit of data I have experienced in my scientific career when someone stood up and showed significant heritability for pimping behaviour. If there is one take-home message, it is that you don't have individual genes for pimping behaviour or other sorts of antisocial behaviour. The idea is that there is a genetic contribution to the basic emotional circuitry which makes antisocial behaviour more or less likely. There is a genetic contribution to the functional integrity of the amygdala from this story, and this determines how well you socialize or not. Others have argued that psychopathy might be due to childhood abuse or some other form of environmental factor. There is definitely environmental impact on the level of antisocial behaviour. However, childhood abuse leads to a child that is highly emotional, not one with reduced emotional responding. As yet there is no social cause that could give rise to the primary emotional deficit in psychopathy. Perhaps, there will be an animal parenting model that will show that a specific type of parenting can give rise to reduced emotional responding, but this has not been documented yet. Adverse environmental circumstances increase the stress response and basic emotional responding throughout the lifespan.

Adolphs: It is an intriguing story, but I had one problem with your hypothesis that it is specifically the amygdala rather than the orbitofrontal cortex that is implicated in psychopathic behaviour. How do you account for the lesion data? There seems to be no evidence that lesions of the amygdala result in any of the constellation of symptoms that you listed, whereas the frontal cortex does show quite a broad spectrum of them.

Blair: The orbitofrontal cortex data are beautiful in that they demonstrate that psychopathy cannot be explained in terms of an orbitofrontal cortex lesion. If orbitofrontal cortex is lesioned, you see an individual prone to reactive aggression and temper tantrums if you see antisocial behaviour. Many patients don't show any problems at all. There has never been a case that I know of that shows heightened levels of instrumental, goal directed aggression. Goal-directed aggression, such as mugging someone for their wallet, is a phenomenon unique to psychopathy. Reactive aggression, irritability, is not. That is why I described the children with bipolar disorder. Childhood bipolar disorder does appear similar in terms of functional impairment to patients with orbitofrontal cortex dysfunction. Both children with bipolar disorder and patients with orbitofrontal cortex dysfunction show problems with socially inappropriate behaviour and pervasive problems in expression recognition. Incidentally, orbitofrontal cortex is not necessary for aversive conditioning and passive avoidance learning. Patients with orbitofrontal cortex lesions do not fail these tasks. Nor, for that matter, do children with bipolar disorder. However, amygdala lesions in animals or humans lead to profound problems in these tasks. Functional impairment is very similar between amygdala lesion cases and individuals with psychopathy. The difference is the amygdala lesion patients are not showing antisocial behaviour. Typically these are lesions in adulthood when they are picked up. We know that the amygdala allows us to learn about the valence of a particular object, but it doesn't store the valence of an object.

Adolphs: Your prediction would therefore be that if you had developmental-onset amygdala lesions, then you would see real life antisocial disorders.

Blair: Yes, but we need to be careful here. It's important to make reference to social circumstances. Although I do not believe there is empirical support for a social explanation of the emotional problems seen in psychopathy, there is considerable impact of social variables on the full behavioural manifestation of the disorder. Psychopathy is a highly class-based disorder and is uncommon in middle or upper class individuals on the basis of the current diagnosis. However, I don't think that the emotional problems are under-represented in individuals of higher socio-economic status (SES) levels. I could be a psychopath and never respond to a sad or fearful face, but because I make money in an alternative way I don't have to rob people on street corners. To test the lesion prediction, we need to have a patient with an amygdala lesion brought up in an adverse environment—I'd be stunned if that individual wasn't more likely to show antisocial behaviour than a healthy developing individual.

Adolphs: What do you make of the developmental amygdala lesions that David Amaral's group has studied? The behaviour they show is the opposite: they show social phobia.

Blair: You are right: they show social phobia. I would like to take children of individuals with psychopathy at an early age and study them. My position is that social threat circuitry runs through orbitofrontal cortex and down into the brain stem while the amygdala conveys other sorts of threat information. We know that those monkeys have problems with snakes and other sorts of learned threat stimuli. The amygdala is also doing a lot of processing of appetitive stimuli. In the Amaral paradigm, the conspecific enters in an intruder scenario, stares at the lesioned monkey. Another's stare is a social threat stimulus. The regular monkey is getting this threat stimulus but also a lot of appetitive information, and does a contingent response to the approaching conspecific. In the lesioned monkey we see an animal that only has social threat information and none of the appetitive stuff. This may be why it is so terrified. The prediction would be that if I had very young individuals with psychopathy, I might also see a heightened social threat response but not a heightened response to aversive conditioning or snakes and other primary threat stimuli. In fact, we clearly don't see those. What we do know is that they are socially isolated at school, but this isn't surprising given that they are aggressive. It is an interesting prediction, but this study hasn't been done.

Singer: You focused on the visual stimuli of facial expressions. Of course there is also learning from sounds associated with aggression or pain. These do not necessarily activate the amygdala. A facial expression of pain is processed by the insula and anterior cingulate cortex (ACC), and only in 30% of pain studies is general amygdale activity observed. How would you account for all the other possibilities for humans to engage in aversive learning not involving amygdale and not involving visual cues?

Blair: It is much worse than that! There are several forms of punishment-based learning where the amygdala is not involved. For example, animal data show that the amygdala is not necessary for punishment-based stimulus–response learning. The prediction would be that individuals with psychopathy will not be impaired in punishment-based learning that does not involve the amygdala. Certainly, they are unimpaired in punishment based stimulus response learning. There is a lot of information available to learn how to behave. However, this is not the sort of stimulus–reinforcement learning that you need in order to do moral socialization.

Singer: Take for example the example of moral disgust, a function which relies entirely on the insula and not on the amygdala. Would you conclude that sociopaths do not show things like incest taboos?

Blair: No, they appear to be intact for moral disgust judgements. This is conventional in the sense that there is no victim involved, but your brain doesn't treat this in the same way that it treats other conventional items. There will be quite a lot of stuff that is intact. If you met these people you wouldn't be able to pick up their psychopathy immediately. It is not like autism or childhood bipolar disorder. The disorder is subtle in behavioural presentation unless you get in the way of these people when they want something.

Moll: If you think that the amygdala is important for learning associations for harm avoidance, we would expect that psychopaths would have general problems with harm avoidance. They seem to be less risk averse, indeed. But I believe that risk taking is at least partially dissociable from lack of empathy. Would you agree that one component would be lack of empathy itself? If so, I'm wondering if and how this would be explained from the perspective of your proposal?

Blair: Risk taking is a separate issue from harm avoidance. I don't know what the data for risk taking in psychopathy is. I don't think there are good data. Risk taking within the Psychopathy Checklist (PCL)-R assessment is indexed by whether the individual changes jobs regularly or whether they have done drugs. It is not indexed by whether they like extreme sports.

Moll: They are more involved in car crashes, for example.

Blair: But then they are using a lot more drugs, which would increase the risk of accidents. If you have an individual with reduced responsiveness to specific types of threat stimuli, then they will be more likely to engage in risky behaviour. I'm assuming that averse responses to high speed have a contribution from the amygdala.

Moll: I wonder if avoiding harm would be correlated with antisocial behaviour, at least with Factor 2 of PCL scores.

Blair: I am not sure there is a good enough index of harm avoidance for us to study it. There are studies reporting comparable levels of harm avoidance in psychopathy and comparison individuals (Herpertz et al 2001) but this is from a self-report questionnaire and this is a population known for pathological lying.

Montague: Why it is when the amygdala is lesioned that people don't start committing crimes?

Blair: Most of the cases are adult lesion cases. The amygdala allows you to learn stimulus–reinforcement associations but it doesn't store this information. The amygdala is necessary to learn the valence of objects or actions but it does not store this information.

Montague: So if I had an intact amygdala until 18 and then had a cardiac event lesioning the amygdala, I will have already stored the way to behave.

Blair: Yes, you would regard moral transgressions as bad and function accordingly.

Montague: It might be worth looking for psychopathy in CEOs who are driven by making money and run over the environment and people around them, and so on.

Blair: I am not doing this sort of work, but Paul Babiak does exactly this (Babiak and Hare 2006). There was a study by Gordon et al (2004) who looked at an undergraduate population. They showed a correlation between psychopathy personality and reduced amygdala response to facial expressions.

Adolphs: I still have the problem that amygdala lesions in humans don't seem to lead to psychopathic behaviour, including ones that are presumably developmental amygdala lesions. People tend to go in the other direction, and people even end up getting taken advantage of.

Montague: This happens in amyotrophic lateral sclerosis, where people routinely develop 'nice guy syndrome'. People will often comfort the doctor as she gives them ever more grim information on successive visits. We did some social exchange games with these people, discovered that if we did the threatening face paradigm, these patients resemble amygdala lesion patients. They don't see threat, and the degree to which they don't see threat seems to scale with this nice guy effect.

Blair: The problem is that there is no neuropsychological model of psychopathy—no brain lesion, whether of frontal cortex or the amygdala, in child or adulthood, that leads to a behavioural syndrome like psychopathy. Some orbitofrontal cortex lesion cases do show aggression. However, their aggression is reactive not instrumental. With respect to individual neuropsychological functions, orbitofrontal cortex lesions are associated with problems in decision making and general problems with expression recognition. These problems are also seen in childhood bipolar disorder. Children with bipolar disorder also show reactive aggression. In other words, orbitofrontal cortex lesion cases may be an applicable neuropsychological model for childhood bipolar disorder even if they are not for psychopathy. Patients with amygdala lesions, but not patients with orbitofrontal cortex lesions, show problems in aversive conditioning, startle reflex augmentation by visual threat primes, passive avoidance learning and fearful expression recognition. So do individuals with psychopathy. In short, the functional impairments associated with amygdala dysfunction are also seen in individuals with psychopathy even if amygdala lesions alone do not inevitably lead to psychopathy.

References

Babiak P, Hare RD 2006 Snakes in suits. Regan Books, in press
Gordon HL, Baird AA, End A 2004 Functional differences among those high and low on a trait measure of psychopathy. Biological Psychiatry 56:516–521
Herpertz SC, Werth U, Lukas G et al 2001 Emotion in criminal offenders with psychopathy and borderline personality disorder. Arch Gen Psychiatry 58:737–745

Looking at other people: mechanisms for social perception revealed in subjects with focal amygdala damage

Ralph Adolphs

Division of Humanities and Social Sciences and Division of Biology, California Institute of Technology, Pasadena, CA 91125, USA

Abstract. How does the presence of socially relevant information in the environment influence our perception and judgment of other people? We have investigated how we direct our gaze to other people's faces, how we use specific features from faces to make social judgments about the presumed internal states of others, and how these mechanisms are disrupted following pathology. Studies of patients with damage to the amygdala have demonstrated a specific impairment in the ability to direct gaze towards, and to use information from, the eyes in others' faces. This basic impairment may explain the deficient recognition of basic emotions and deficient social judgment seen in such patients. Ongoing studies in our laboratory examine face-to-face social interactions with real people in an attempt to link the above impairments in the laboratory to the dysfunctional social cognition seen in everyday life.

2006 Empathy and Fairness. Wiley, Chichester (Novartis Foundation Symposium 278) p 146–164

No one would deny that much of primate social behaviour is modulated by processing that is best described as 'emotional', both in the sense that aspects of emotions (such as psychophysiological responses and conscious feelings of an emotion) accompany the processing, and in the sense that brain structures known to subserve emotions are engaged. Indeed, ever since Darwin's seminal book, *The expression of the emotions in man and animals*, we have included emotional expression as a key component of social behaviour. We smile and frown at one another, and such non-verbal social communication forms much of the topic of 'social neuroscience'.

What are the mechanisms behind our ability to recognize others' emotional expressions (Fig. 1)? One account has proposed that emotional responses in the viewer to the perceived expressions of another person may share aspects of the emotion displayed by the person who is being observed. This idea, that we simulate aspects of other people's emotions in order to derive information about their

146

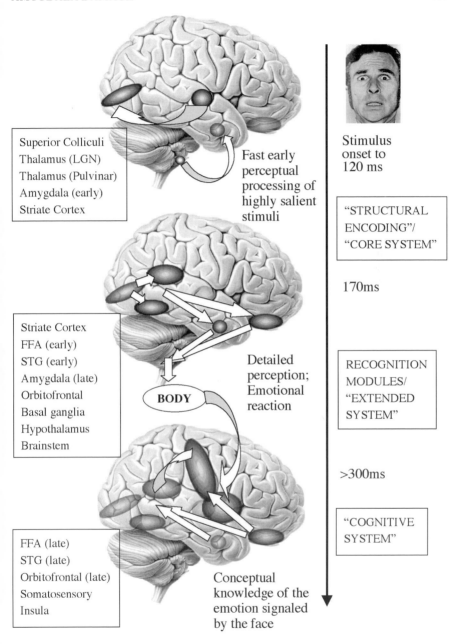

Superior Colliculi
Thalamus (LGN)
Thalamus (Pulvinar)
Amygdala (early)
Striate Cortex

Fast early perceptual processing of highly salient stimuli

Stimulus onset to 120 ms

"STRUCTURAL ENCODING"/ "CORE SYSTEM"

170ms

Striate Cortex
FFA (early)
STG (early)
Amygdala (late)
Orbitofrontal
Basal ganglia
Hypothalamus
Brainstem

BODY

Detailed perception; Emotional reaction

RECOGNITION MODULES/ "EXTENDED SYSTEM"

>300ms

"COGNITIVE SYSTEM"

FFA (late)
STG (late)
Orbitofrontal (late)
Somatosensory
Insula

Conceptual knowledge of the emotion signaled by the face

FIG. 1.   Initial model of how the amygdala and somatosensory cortices could work together in simulation-based recognition of emotion from facial expressions. On the left are indicated some of the structures shown in the middle on views of a brain; on the right are indicated some of the processes to which they roughly correspond. The figure begins with the onset of the stimulus, a facial expression of emotion, at the top, and progresses through perception to final recognition of the emotion at the bottom. Note that the figure omits many structures and connections in order to provide a schematic overview. Reproduced from Adolphs (2002).

internal state, has both sensory and motor aspects to it. We can feel another person's emotions; but we can also engage some of the motor and premotor representations that would be required to produce the emotional expression seen in the other person. Originally articulated by Titchener, Lipps and others (Lipps 1907), this idea has received considerable recent attention with the discovery of 'mirror neurons' that respond both to one's own actions as well as to those of a conspecific, and the discovery that somatic mapping structures in the brain are activated both when we feel an emotion and observe another person express it (Blakemore & Decety 2001, Gallese 2003, Gallese & Goldman 1999, Rizzolatti et al 2001).

There are now several studies indicating that the observation of another person's emotional state recruits structures like the insula (Jackson et al 2005, Singer et al 2004), an interoceptive somatosensory cortex also involved in representing our own somatic states. Interestingly, the insula has been hypothesized (Craig 2002, Damasio 1999) and recently shown (Critchley et al 2004) to be associated with the conscious experience of our own body state. This suggests that our knowledge of another person's emotional state through simulation of their presumed somatic state relies on a simulation that is explicit, in the sense of providing conscious access to the emotion that is being simulated. That is, the simulation mechanism through which we infer another person's emotion is empathic: it involves actually feeling (aspects of) the emotion of the other person.

In one study from our laboratory, we found evidence supporting a role for simulation in emotion recognition (Adolphs et al 2000). In a lesion study of 108 patients with focal brain damage, it was found that lesions in right somatosensory cortices (including insula) were associated with impairments in the ability to recognize emotion from other people's facial expressions. One interpretation of the findings was as follows: in order to trigger an image of the somatosensory state associated with an emotion, we use structures that link perception of the stimulus (the facial expression seen) to a somatic response (or directly to the representation thereof). One route for triggering such an emotional response to viewing another person's expression in the first place would be structures such as the amygdala, long known to associate emotionally salient sensory stimuli with emotional responses. Below I review the research findings that support such a mechanism for the amygdala; in the subsequent section I describe our latest findings that suggest an alternative explanation.

Fear recognition and the amygdala

Several lesion studies (Adolphs et al 1994, Anderson & Phelps 2000, Anderson et al 2000, Calder et al 1996, Young et al 1996), complemented by functional imaging studies (Breiter et al 1996, Morris et al 1996, Whalen et al 2001), have demonstrated that the human amygdala is critical for normal judgments about the internal states of others from viewing pictures of their facial expressions. Some studies have found a disproportionately severe impairment in recognizing fear (Adolphs et al 1995, Anderson & Phelps 2000, Broks et al 1998, Calder et al 1996, Sprengelmeyer et al 1999), whereas others have found evidence for a broader or more variable impairment in recognizing multiple emotions of negative valence in the face, including fear, anger, disgust, and sadness (Adolphs 1999, Adolphs et al 1999, Schmolck & Squire 2001) (Siebert et al 2003). Across the majority of studies, impairments in recognition of emotion have been found despite an often normal ability to discriminate perceptually among the same stimuli. Many patients with bilateral amygdala damage perform in the normal range on the Benton Face Matching Task (Benton et al 1983), in which subjects are asked to match different views of the same, unfamiliar person's face, and they also perform normally in discriminating subtle changes in facial expression, even for facial expressions that they are nonetheless unable to recognize (Adolphs & Tranel 2000, Adolphs et al 1998).

We have studied in detail a rare subject, SM, who has been especially informative because of the specificity of both her lesion and her impairment (Adolphs & Tranel 2000, Tranel & Hyman 1990). SM is a 40 year old woman who has complete bilateral amygdala damage resulting from a rare disease (Urbach-Wiethe disease; Hofer 1973) (Fig. 2). On a series of tasks, she shows a relatively disproportionate impairment in recognizing the intensity of fear from faces alone, and a lesser impairment also in recognizing the intensity of related emotions such as surprise and anger (Adolphs et al 1994) (Fig. 3).

A further role for the amygdala in processing aspects of faces comes from studies of the interaction between facial emotion and eye gaze. The direction of eye gaze in other individuals' faces is an important source of information about their emotional state, intention, and likely future behaviour. Eye gaze is a key social signal in many species (Emery 2000), especially apes and humans, whose white sclera makes the pupil more easily visible and permits better discrimination of gaze. Human viewers make preferential fixations onto the eye region of others' faces (Janik et al 1978), a behaviour that appears early in development and may contribute to the socioemotional impairments seen in developmental disorders like autism (Baron-Cohen 1995). Eyes signal important information about emotional states, and there is evidence from functional imaging studies that at least some of this processing recruits the amygdala (Baron-Cohen et al 1999, Kawashima et al 1999, Wicker et al 2003). The interaction between facial emotion and direction of eye gaze has been explored only very recently. It was found that direct gaze facilitated processing of approach-oriented emotions such as anger, whereas averted gaze facilitated the processing of avoidance-oriented emotions such as fear (Adams & Kleck 2003), and that this processing facilitation correlated with increased activation of the amygdala in a functional imaging study (Adams et al 2003).

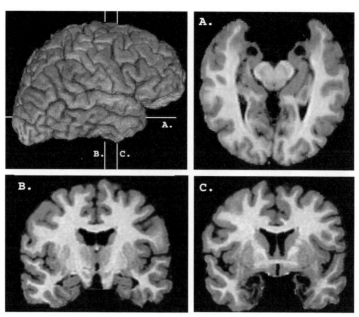

FIG. 2.   Neuroanatomy of SM046. Shown on the top left is a 3D reconstruction of SM's brain from magnetic resonance images, showing the planes of section of the other cuts. The symmetrical region of low signal in the anteromedial temporal lobe is due to calcification and atrophy of tissue within the entire amygdala as well as anterior entorhinal cortex. The damage resulted from a rare genetic disease, Urbach-Wiethe disease.

FIG. 3.   Bilateral amygdala damage impairs recognition of multiple negative emotions. While subject SM shows a disproportionate impairment in the ability to recognize fear, most subjects with bilateral amygdala damage show broader impairments in multiple negatively valenced emotions. Raw rating scores of facial expressions of emotion are shown from seven normal controls, from 16 brain-damaged controls with no amygdala damage, and from eight subjects with bilateral amygdala damage. The emotional stimuli (36 faces; six each of the six basic emotions indicated) are ordered on the y-axis according to their perceived similarity (stimuli perceived to be similar, e.g. two happy faces, or a happy and a surprised faces, are adjacent; stimuli perceived to be dissimilar, e.g. happy and sad faces, are distant). The six emotion labels on which subjects rated the faces are displayed on the x-axis. Greyscale brightness encodes the mean rating given to each face by a group of subjects, as indicated in the scale. Thus, a darker line would indicate a lower mean rating than a brighter line for a given face; and a thin bright line for a given emotion category would indicate that few stimuli of that emotion received a high rating, whereas a thick bright line would indicate that many or all stimuli within that emotion category received high ratings. Data from subjects with bilateral amygdala damage indicate abnormally low ratings of negative emotions (thinner bright bands across any horizontal position corresponding to an expression of a negative emotion). From Adolphs et al (1999), © Elsevier Science Publishers.

The amygdala's role is not limited to making judgments about basic emotions, but includes a role in making social judgments. This fact was already suggested by earlier studies in non-human primates (Kling & Brothers 1992, Kluver & Bucy 1937, Rosvold et al 1954) which demonstrated impaired social behaviour following amygdala damage. They have been corroborated in recent times by studies in monkeys with more selective amygdala lesions, and by using more sophisticated

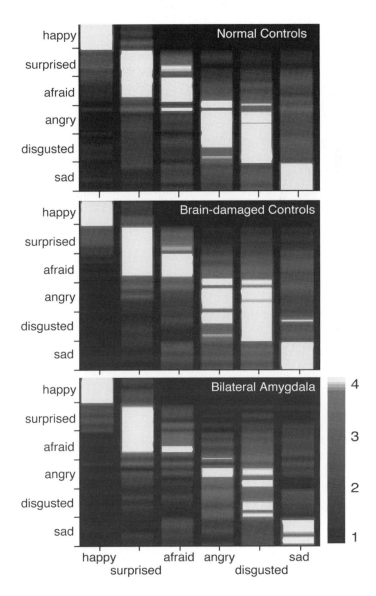

ways of assessing social behaviour (Emery & Amaral 1999, Emery et al 2001), and they have been shown now also in humans. Building on these findings, some recent studies suggest a general role for the amygdala in so-called 'theory of mind' abilities: the collection of abilities whereby we attribute internal mental states, intentions, desires and emotions to other people (Baron-Cohen et al 2000, Fine et al 2001). Related to this, the amygdala shows differential habituation of activation to faces of people of another race (Hart et al 2000), and amygdala activation has been found to correlate with race stereotypes of which the viewer may be unaware (Phelps et al 2000). However, the amygdala's role in processing information about race is still unclear: other brain regions, in extrastriate visual cortex, are also activated differentially as a function of race (Golby et al 2001) and lesions of the amygdala do not appear to impair race judgments (Phelps et al 2003).

The above findings supported the simulation view of how emotional expressions might be recognized. Visual cortices in the temporal lobe would be involved in perceptual processing of facial features, would then convey a perceptual representation of the face to the basolateral amygdala, which in turn would associate it with its emotional response, likely effected by a variety of amygdala nuclei and corresponding to changes in a number of measures. One such change would be the somatic response triggered by the central nucleus of the amygdala: changes in autonomic tone, for example. These emotional responses, in turn, would be perceived and represented in somatosensory cortices including the insula, and would form the direct substrate for sharing the observed person's feeling of the emotion (Fig. 1).

A new view of the role of the amygdala in emotion recognition

This account of how we might infer another's emotional state via simulation (Goldman & Sripada 2005) turned out to be an incomplete picture. A more recent study gave the surprising finding that the amygdala comes into play in a more abstract, and earlier, processing component (Adolphs et al 2005). Amygdala damage was found to impair the ability to use information from a diagnostic facial feature—the eye region of the face. Following amygdala damage, the eye region of faces was no longer used effectively by the viewer in order to discriminate fear. These findings were consistent with other results showing amygdala activation to fearful eyes (Morris et al 2002), or only to the briefly presented whites of eyes (Whalen et al 2004).

The experiment that demonstrated this finding used a new technique, called 'bubbles', in which small portions of an image of a face were revealed to viewers. For example, on a particular trial, a viewer might see only the ear of an underlying face, or perhaps part of the cheek and part of the forehead. Some quick reflection immediately suggests that not all regions of the face would be equally informative about the emotion: seeing part of an ear does not distinguish emotions, whereas seeing part of the eyes or the mouth is much more discriminative in that regard. One can take advantage of this fact using a procedure similar to reverse correlation. When shown these randomly revealed pieces of faces, subjects are asked to judge the emotion. Those trials they get correct are all summed, and we now subtract all those trials (i.e. those pieces of faces) that they get incorrect. This procedure (or its continuous analogue, regressing performance accuracy on the regions of the face that are revealed in each trial), generates a so-called 'classification image' that denotes the regions of the face on the basis of which subjects are able to discriminate the emotion.

Perhaps not too surprisingly, the classification image for discriminating fear from happiness (the particular discrimination we used in our experiment) prominently shows the eyes and the mouth. However, when the same experiment was conducted in subject SM mentioned earlier, who has bilateral amygdala damage, the classification image did not contain as much of the eyes. In fact the impaired use of visual information from the face in subject SM was very specific: she failed to make use of high spatial frequency information from the eye region of faces (Fig. 4).

In fact, the deficit was even more basic than that: the reason that information about the eye region was not used effectively in subject SM was because the eye region was not fixated in the first place (Fig. 5). A second experiment measured viewers' eye movements as they judged the emotion shown in facial expressions. While healthy individuals spend a lot of time fixating the eye region of faces, subject SM failed to do so. Thus, her impaired use of visual information about the eye region of the face was likely derivative to an impaired ability to allocate visual attention and fixate the eye region in the first place. Her brain did not possess the mechanism to decide which regions of a face to explore preferentially in order to glean relevant information about the emotion.

The above findings could provide the basis for impaired fear recognition following amygdala damage. Since the eye region of faces is most important in order to distinguish fear from other emotions, and since SM fails to fixate and make use of information about the eye region of faces, her impaired fear recognition apparently results from her impaired fixation of the eyes in faces. A final experiment tested this interpretation directly: we instructed SM to direct her gaze onto the eyes of other people's faces, and found that this manipulation temporarily allowed her to generate a normal performance on a fear recognition task in which she was otherwise severely impaired (Fig. 6).

It is worth noting two key further results from this study. First, SM failed to fixate the eyes in any face, not just facial expressions of fear. In fact, she simply failed to explore faces in general, which included a failure to direct her gaze towards the eye region. Similarly, the abnormal use of information from the eye

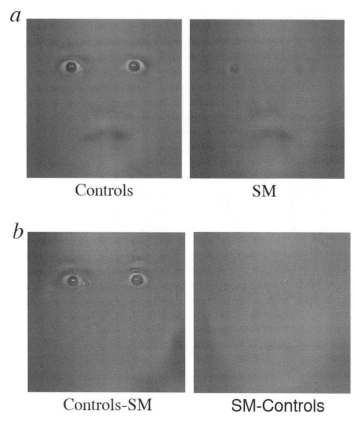

FIG. 4.   Impaired ability to use information from the eye region of the face in subject SM. Using a new technique ('bubbles'), it was found that controls benefit substantially in their ability to discriminate fear when they are shown the eye region of the face, whereas SM does not. (A) effective information used by controls (left) and SM (right) to discriminate fearful from happy images of sparsely revealed faces. (B) difference images showing which facial information is used more by controls than by SM (left) or by SM than by controls (right). Data from Adolphs et al (2005), © MacMillan Press.

region held for happy faces as well as for fearful faces. So the impairment in use of information from, and fixation onto, the eyes in faces was general for faces. The reason that this general impairment resulted in a relatively specific impairment in fear recognition was just because the eye region of the face was in fact the most diagnostic for signalling fear, rather than other emotions. Given the recognition tasks we used, this resulted in a severe impairment in recognizing fear, but not in recognizing other emotions. (Interestingly, unpublished data indicate that the same subject does fixate the eye region when the faces are shown inverted. So, while the

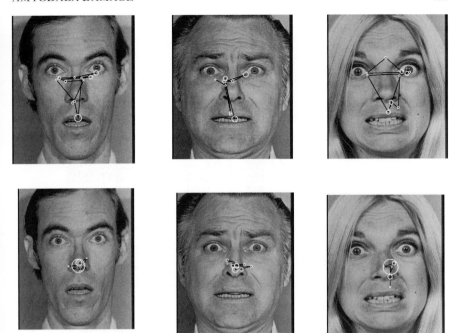

FIG. 5. Impaired spontaneous fixations on the face in subject SM. When viewing faces without any specific instructions about fixation, SM failed to explore the faces with her gaze, and failed to fixate the eye regions of the face. Top panel: three sample face stimuli with overlaid fixations (white circles) and saccades (black lines) given by a normal control. Bottom panel: data from subject SM. Data from Adolphs et al (2005), © MacMillan Press.

brain does not need to know that the face is showing fear in order for the impaired eye fixations to occur, it apparently does need to know that the stimulus is a face; the impairment in fixation does not seem to generalize to objects other than faces, including inverted faces).

A second point worth noting is that the explicit instruction to fixate the eyes in faces, while rescuing SM's impaired recognition of fear, did so only transiently (as long as that block of the experiment lasted). When later asked to view faces, SM spontaneously reverted to her lack of exploration of the face, and once again showed impaired fear recognition. One reason that the improvement was not more permanent may well be that SM was not given additional information about her impairment. She was unaware that she failed to fixate the eyes, as she was unaware that her performance in fear recognition was impaired. This raises further questions: why did she not ask about her performance, why did she not notice that she failed to fixate the eyes? I believe that these questions point towards a broader

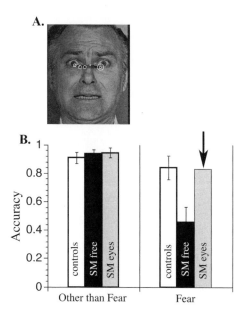

FIG. 6. Rescue of impaired fear recognition with instructed fixations onto the eyes. (A) Despite her lack of spontaneous fixations to the eye region of faces, SM was able to fixate those regions when instructed explicitly to do so. (B) This manipulation changed her otherwise impaired recognition of fear ('SM free' in the graph on the right) to an essentially normal performance accuracy ('SM eyes', bar denoted by the arrow). Data from Adolphs et al (2005), © MacMillan Press.

interpretation of the impairment. SM, as a result of damage to the amygdala, lacked a normal mechanism to explore the environment. One aspect of such an impairment was a failure to fixate the eyes in faces, to explore them normally with one's gaze. Another aspect of the impairment was a failure to question what was going on in the experiment in any way, or to monitor one's own performance during it. In both cases, there remains a passive ability to process sensory information, but the instrumental component of seeking out such information in the first place has been severely compromised.

Conclusions

These new data indicate that the amygdala comes into play much earlier than initially thought, and in a more abstract way that is not specialized for recognizing fear as such. It appears to be specialized for seeking out potentially salient social information in the first place, by directing our gaze and visual attention to certain regions of faces that should be explored in more detail. It may be that this role extends beyond faces to a broader role in exploration of the social environment generally (Sander et al 2003), as the above discussion suggests, similar to earlier proposals that the amygdala serves to detect potentially important stimuli about which more information must be gathered (Whalen 1999).

While the amygdala thus appears to be involved in strategies for picking up relevant social information from the environment through exploration, it may well also be involved in triggering somatic emotional responses to the stimuli thus processed. That is, the new role in active exploration and attention allocation does not preclude the earlier ideas that the amygdala could provide the initial input for simulation-based mechanisms of emotion recognition. One possibility might be that the two aspects of amygdala function are effected via different amygdala nuclei, an idea that would require better spatial resolution in studies of the human amygdala than is typically possible in lesion experiments, although to some extent imaging experiments and intracranial electrophysiological studies could circumvent this difficulty.

Acknowledgements

Supported by grants from the National Institute of Mental Health, the Pfeiffer Research Foundation, the Cure Autism Now Foundation, and the National Alliance for Autism Research.

References

Adams RB, Kleck RE 2003 Perceived gaze direction and the processing of facial displays of emotion. Psychological Science 14:644–647
Adams RB, Gordon HL, Baird AA, Ambady N, Kleck RE 2003 Effects of gaze on amygdala sensitivity to anger and fear faces. Science 300:1536
Adolphs R 1999 The human amygdala and emotion. The Neuroscientist 5:125–137
Adolphs R 2002 Recognizing emotion from facial expressions: psychological and neurological mechanisms. Behav Cogn Neurosci Rev 1:21–61
Adolphs R, Tranel D 2000 Emotion recognition and the human amygdala. In: Aggleton JP (ed), The amygdala. A functional analysis. Oxford University Press, New York, p 587–630
Adolphs R, Tranel D, Damasio H, Damasio A 1994 Impaired recognition of emotion in facial expressions following bilateral damage to the human amygdala. Nature 372:669–672
Adolphs R, Tranel D, Damasio H, Damasio AR 1995 Fear and the human amygdala. J Neurosci 15:5879–5892
Adolphs R, Tranel D, Damasio AR 1998 The human amygdala in social judgment. Nature 393:470–474
Adolphs R, Tranel D, Hamann S et al 1999 Recognition of facial emotion in nine subjects with bilateral amygdala damage. Neuropsychologia 37:1111–1117

Adolphs R, Damasio H, Tranel D, Cooper G, Damasio AR 2000 A role for somatosensory cortices in the visual recognition of emotion as revealed by 3-D lesion mapping. J Neurosci 20:2683–2690

Adolphs R, Gosselin F, Buchanan TW, Tranel D, Schyns PG, Damasio A 2005 A mechanism for impaired fear recognition after amygdala damage. Nature 433:68–72

Anderson AK, Phelps EA 2000 Expression without recognition: contributions of the human amygdala to emotional communication. Psychological Science 11:106–111

Anderson AK, Spencer DD, Fulbright RK, Phelps EA 2000 Contribution of the anteromedial temporal lobes to the evaluation of facial emotion. Neuropsychology 14:526–536

Baron-Cohen S 1995 Mindblindness: an essay on autism and theory of mind. MIT Press, Cambridge, MA

Baron-Cohen S, Ring HA, Wheelwright S et al 1999 Social intelligence in the normal and autistic brain: an fMRI study. Eur J Neurosci 11:1891–1898

Baron-Cohen S, Ring HA, Bullmore ET, Wheelwright S, Ashwin C, Williams SCR 2000 The amygdala theory of autism. Neurosci Biobehav Rev 24:355–364

Benton AL, Hamsher K, Varney NR, Spreen O 1983 Contributions to neuropsychological assessment. Oxford University Press, New York

Blakemore S-J, Decety J 2001 From the perception of action to the understanding of intention. Nat Rev Neurosci 2:561–568

Breiter HC, Etcoff NL, Whalen PJ et al 1996 Response and habituation of the human amygdala during visual processing of facial expression. Neuron 17:875–887

Broks P, Young AW, Maratos EJ et al 1998 Face processing impairments after encephalitis: amygdala damage and recognition of fear. Neuropsychologia 36:59–70

Calder AJ, Young AW, Rowland D, Perrett DI, Hodges JR, Etcoff NL 1996 Facial emotion recognition after bilateral amygdala damage: differentially severe impairment of fear. Cognitive Neuropsychology 13:699–745

Craig AD 2002 How do you feel? Interoception: the sense of the physiological condition of the body. Nat Rev Neurosci 3:655–666

Critchley HD, Wiens S, Rotshtein P, Oehman A, Dolan RJ 2004 Neural systems supporting interoceptive awareness. Nat Neurosci 7:189–195

Damasio AR 1999 The feeling of what happens: body and emotion in the making of consciousness. Harcourt Brace, New York

Emery NJ 2000 The eyes have it: the neuroethology, function and evolution of social gaze. Neurosci Biobehav Rev 24:581–604

Emery NJ, Amaral DG 1999 The role of the amygdala in primate social cognition. In: Lane RD, Nadel L (eds), Cognitive neuroscience of emotion. Oxford University Press, Oxford p 156–191

Emery NJ, Capitanio JP, Mason WA, Machado CJ, Mendoza SP, Amaral DG 2001 The effects of bilateral lesions of the amygdala on dyadic social interactions in rhesus monkeys. Behav Neurosci 115:515–544

Fine C, Lumsden J, Blair RJR 2001 Dissociation between 'theory of mind' and executive functions in a patient with early left amygdala damage. Brain 124:287–298

Gallese V 2003 The manifold nature of interpersonal relations: the quest for a common mechanism. Philos Trans R Soc Lond B Biol Sci 358:517–528

Gallese V, Goldman A 1999 Mirror neurons and the simulation theory of mind reading. Trends Cogn Sci 2:493–500

Golby AJ, Gabrieli JDE, Chiao JY, Eberhardt JL 2001 Differential responses in the fusiform region to same-race and other-race faces. Nat Neurosci 4:845–850

Goldman AI, Sripada CS 2005 Simulationist models of face-based emotion recognition. Cognition 94:193–213

Hart AJ, Whalen PJ, Shin LM, McInerney SC, Fischer H, Rauch SL 2000 Differential response in the human amygdala to racial outgroup vs ingroup face stimuli. NeuroReport 11: 2351–2355

Hofer P-A 1973 Urbach-Wiethe disease: a review. Acta Derm Venerol 53:5–52

Jackson PL, Meltzoff AN, Decety J 2005 How do we perceive the pain of others? A window into the neural processes involved in empathy. Neuroimage 24:771–779

Janik SW, Wellens AR, Goldberg ML, Dell'Osso LF 1978 Eyes as the center of focus in the visual examination of human faces. Percept Mot Skills 47:857–858

Kawashima R, Sugiura M, Kato T et al 1999 The human amygdala plays an important role in gaze monitoring. Brain 122:779–783

Kling AS, Brothers LA 1992 The amygdala and social behavior. In: Aggleton JP (ed), The amygdala: neurobiological aspects of emotion, memory, and mental dysfunction. Wiley-Liss, New York

Kluver H, Bucy PC 1937 'Psychic blindness' and other symptoms following bilateral temporal lobectomy in rhesus monkeys. Am J Physiol 119:352–353

Lipps T 1907 Psychologische Untersuchungen. Engelman, Leipzig

Morris JS, Frith CD, Perrett DI et al 1996 A differential neural response in the human amygdala to fearful and happy facial expressions. Nature 383:812–815

Morris JS, deBonis M, Dolan RJ 2002 Human amygdala responses to fearful eyes. Neuroimage 17:214–222

Phelps EA, O'Connor KJ, Cunningham WA et al 2000 Performance on indirect measures of race evaluation predicts amygdala activation. J Cogn Neurosci 12:729–738

Phelps EA, Cannistraci CJ, Cunningham WA 2003 Intact performance on an indirect measure of race bias following amygdala damage. Neuropsychologia 41:203–209

Rizzolatti G, Fogassi L, Gallese V 2001 Neurophysiological mechanisms underlying the understanding and imitation of action. Nat Rev Neurosci 2:661–670

Rosvold HE, Mirsky AF, Pribram K 1954 Influence of amygdalectomy on social behavior in monkeys. J Comp Physiol Psychol 47:173–178

Sander D, Grafman J, Zalla T 2003 The human amygdala: an evolved sytem for relevance detection. Rev Neurosci 14:303–316

Schmolck H, Squire LR 2001 Impaired perception of facial emotions following bilateral damage to the anterior temporal lobe. Neuropsychology 15:30–38

Siebert M, Markowitsch HJ, Bartel P 2003 Amygdala, affect and cognition: evidence from 10 patients with Urbach-Wiethe disease. Brain 126:2627–2637

Singer T, Seymour B, O'Doherty J, Kaube H, Dolan RJ, Frith CD 2004 Empathy for pain involves the affective but not sensory components of pain. Science 303:1157–1162

Sprengelmeyer R, Young AW, Schroeder U et al 1999 Knowing no fear. Proc R Soc London Series B 266:2451–2456

Tranel D, Hyman BT 1990 Neuropsychological correlates of bilateral amygdale damage. Arch Neurol 47:349–355

Whalen PJ 1999 Fear, vigilance, and ambiguity: initial neuroimaging studies of the human amygdala. Current Directions in Psychological Science 7:177–187

Whalen PJ, Shin LM, McInerney SC, Fischer H, Wright CI, Rauch SL 2001 A functional MRI study of human amygdala responses to facial expressions of fear versus anger. Emotion 1: 70–83

Whalen PJ, Kagan J, Cook RG et al 2004 Human amygdala responsivity to masked fearful eye whites. Science 306:2061

Wicker B, Perrett DI, Baron-Cohen S, Decety J 2003 Being the target of another's emotion: a PET study. Neuropsychologia 41:139–146

Young AW, Hellawell DJ, Van de Wal C, Johnson M 1996 Facial expression processing after amygdalotomy. Neuropsychologia 34:31–39

DISCUSSION

C Frith: You talked about fear as an expression. When you look at other facial expressions, are there different bits of the face that you should look at for each expression?

Adolphs: The finding was that this subject with amygdala damage fails to make use of the eye region for all facial expressions. The reason she is impaired mostly for fear is that because the eyes are the most diagnostic feature for fear and not other emotions. You can apply the same for other emotions. Smith et al (2005) did exactly this. They looked at all the six different emotions and used this bubbles method. For happiness, the smile is most important, for disgust the furrowed brow is key, and so on. There are particular features of faces that are the most informative for discriminating particular emotional expressions in this task. We need to remember that this is a discrimination task, in which subjects are asked to discriminate among different emotional expressions.

C Frith: Is the amygdala involved in directing you to the right part of the face for all these different expressions?

Adolphs: We haven't tested this. All the data I showed related just to the contrast between fear and happiness.

Hauser: What was striking about your quick skim through moral memories is that there was virtually nothing about omissions.

Adolphs: Mostly they are about actions. This is an important distinction.

Hauser: I have a question about the nature of facial expressions, and what they are doing. There was a view that came out of the early ethological literature that was against the commonly shared view of the nature of facial expressions which is that they are information bearing. This alternative view came from the game theory literature, arguing that communicative signals are about manipulating the behaviour of others. Is there any evidence that people with amygdala damage or psychopathy, when they communicate, are selectively doing different things about their expressions when they give them? I'm thinking in terms of the delivery of the expressions, not the recognition.

Adolphs: We have tried to look at this, but it is much harder to measure. I am not aware of any studies looking at the production end of this. You would need some kind of naturalistic situation to elicit the valid production. You'd want to measure facial expressions to some complex social situation. People have measured production of facial expressions in response to overt command, for instance the study by Anderson and Phelps (Anderson & Phelps 2000).

Hauser: I'm thinking of a situation where there is an opportunity to help. The interpretation is that the expression I give is conveying my empathy towards you, but perhaps it is to manipulate the behaviour of the individual in need of help. If you were a psychopath you wouldn't do that because there is no intent to help.

Blair: This isn't properly documented at all, but if you were going to go for a cue, you probably would use the reduced production of emotional expressions in the psychopathic individuals. The paradigm to do would be the Fridlund study, where you manipulate the degree to which the person thinks they are in a social environment, and you show that the amount of smiling behaviour to a cartoon is proportional to the proximity of the audience. I don't know whether it is manipulation of a releasing condition for the behaviour, but facial expressions of emotions are a communicatory act. It's only worth doing a communicatory act when there is someone to communicate to. If I was going to make a prediction, it would be that psychopaths have somewhat muted responses.

C Frith: We were at a meeting recently on embodied cognition. There are people out there who are studying the production side, although not in these abnormal cases. Janet Bavelas is currently conducting a study comparing people telling a story into a tape recorder, over the telephone or face to face: there are dramatic increases in facial expressions and even changes in syntax as the interaction with the listener increases.

Montague: What brought this patient you described into the clinic in the first place? And what have you now concluded is wrong with her, given that you can instruct her to look at the eyes and she is indistinguishable in task performance from controls? What is it that the amygdala lesion has done to her? Is it inappropriate visual search?

Adolphs: She is suffering from a dermatological disease called lipoid proteinosis. There are other aspects to the phenotype, including hoarse voice and abnormal skin healing. The CNS abnormality is not 100%: in half of the cases or so we get mediotemporal calcifications, as in this case. The gene responsible has been identified (Hamada et al 2002).

Montague: So she didn't come in complaining of a cognitive deficit?

Adolphs: No. Her neuropsychological profile is fairly normal. She lives independently and has raised three children. Her maternal behaviour seems entirely normal. She has a network of friends and neighbours. Her social decision making isn't entirely normal, but this is subtle. It is striking how normal she is, though, in her social behaviour.

Montague: And what have you now concluded is wrong with her, given that you can instruct her to look at the eyes and she is indistinguishable in task performance from controls? What is it that the amygdala lesion has done to her? Is it inappropriate visual search?

Adolphs: It is quite surprising: if we instruct her just to look at the eyes, then her face processing then becomes normal and the amygdala seems inessential, and this would be hard to explain.

Montague: You showed an amazing looking graph. It suggests that the amygdala is involved in some sort of processing.

Adolphs: That graph is that performance on that particular task. If you show her facial expressions of fear and ask other kinds of questions, she might still be impaired even if she looks at the eyes. In this task it is sufficient to get information about the eyes to distinguish fear from the other options. When you are telling her to look at the eyes you are doing at least two things. You are making her fixate the eyes, to gain high spatial frequency information about the eye region present at the level of the retina. You are also telling her to allocate visual attention towards the eyes, and you are probably also telling her to process it in some ways.

Gergely: It may have been the autistic study you mentioned where what you see is that people start with the mouth and then they do go to monitor the eyes. So why don't they pick up the information then? Why do you have to first go to the eyes?

Adolphs: Presumably, the time at which the information is available relates to how it is processed. When you process something early on you are biased in some way in terms of how that information is used.

Montague: It is the marginals, I guess. If you sample the eyes first and then on down.

Adolphs: One prediction would be that the shorter we make the stimulus presentation, the more impaired they should become, which seems to be the case.

Sigman: One thing you didn't say is that after she has looked at the eyes, she doesn't if you don't tell her to on subsequent occasions.

Adolphs: Yes, she is unaware of the fact that she has a cognitive impairment. She knows she has amygdala lesions and that is it. We haven't given her extensive feedback so she is relatively unaware of her performance. She is also unaware of the fact that instructing her to look at the eyes changed her performance. When we did the same experiment again she went back to not looking at the eyes.

Singer: Is she saying that it is unpleasant for her to look at the eyes?

Adolphs: There is no evidence to suggest that she has any kind of aversion to looking at the eyes. She did a task where the face came up and the location of the eyes corresponded to the previous location of the fixation spot. There is no faster latency for her looking away from this. She just doesn't know where to look.

Van Lange: You are saying that her social function doesn't seem abnormal. It could be that this is because there are lots of ways of getting information about the emotional state of others. Non-verbal communication is just one of them. Could it be that she is compensating by using other sources of information?

Adolphs: It is critical to keep in mind that the extent to which the social behaviour is normal or not depends on the social environment that the person is placed in. In her own environment, people know she has a brain lesion, so it is an extremely supportive environment. I think the environment is picking up a lot of the slack. People will go out of their way to make friends with her.

Dupoux: You said at the beginning that she had no problem with discriminating stimuli, and could even tell the difference between two kinds of fear. How does she do this if the primary cue is the eyes and she is not looking at them?

Adolphs: In the one experiment where we showed pieces of faces, the discrimination is between fear and happiness. How can she do the task if she can't recognize fear? If it is just a two-alternative task, then she can work out fear by figuring out what is not happy.

Dupoux: I thought initially you said she had excellent discrimination and the only problem was identification?

Adolphs: If you ask her to do a difference task she is normal, yes. In this sort of experiment you see one face at a time and have to match it to different categories.

Call: What would happen if you blocked visual access to the mouth region? Would she go to the eyes?

Adolphs: No. This is what happens in showing pieces of faces. If you just reveal the eyes she doesn't look at them. There is still a sense of an underlying face in these stimuli. The interesting experiment would be to give a blank screen and then just the eyes came up. I imagine she would look at these, since there is nothing else at all salient in the image then.

Blakemore: Is her eye movement pattern normal for non-face stimuli?

Adolphs: To some extent. She explores complex stimuli such as scenes, more so than for faces. She also makes much more normal eye movements when the faces are inverted. It is somehow a deficit specific to faces.

Gallese: If I understood correctly, she fails to look at the eyes, but when she is forced to she can spot a fearful expression from a different one. In contrast, high-functioning autistics don't look at the eyes but can manage to solve the task. We don't know whether this is because they use mouth-related cues or whether they later go to the eyes.

Adolphs: We know that people with autism do not make normal use of the eyes and make exaggerated use of the mouth in order to achieve the same performance accuracy.

Gallese: This would mean that in order to make proficient use of mouth-related cues, you need an intact amygdala. If not, this patient would be normal without being forced to look at the eyes.

Adolphs: I guess so.

Gallese: What about other modalities? If high-functioning autistics are asked to discriminate different emotions on the basis of a sound such as a shout or laugh, how do they do?

Adolphs: We have tried recognition of fear in voices in our patients. Different studies have shown different things. It is only the visual work that has been explored in detail. We don't want to conclude from this work that it is evidence that the amygdala is dysfunctional in autism. These two look different.

Moll: What would you expect if you presented faces very quickly, say during 20 ms, without any masking?

Adolphs: I expect she wouldn't differ in her performance. Normal subjects would show a decrement in their ability to discriminate fear. At the level of the retina they would have available what she has. They wouldn't have high spatial frequency about the eyes, which is specifically the information that she fails to use in that task.

Montague: How does she read the faces of her children?

Adolphs: We haven't tested this. All we know is that she has raised three children. She seems attached to them and is concerned about them.

Montague: Is her processing of high frequency information normal when you test it? Maybe that pathway has degenerated in her retina.

Adolphs: We haven't formally tested that.

Blakemore: Can you get normal people to behave like her? If we fixate on the nose we can still tell what sort of facial expression we are looking at. If you manipulate the attention of normal people to different parts of the face in a distraction task can you get them to behave like her?

Adolphs: The prediction would be that we should be able to.

Brosnan: I am curious about what she perceives as being wrong with her. You haven't told her what is different about her and she didn't know she had brain problems until she had a CT scan. But she obviously knows that she is interesting enough to be travelling to Iowa to get tested on a regular basis.

Adolphs: That is an interesting question. It speaks to a consequence of her amygdala damage. She doesn't know what is important, so she doesn't look at salient regions of the face. She is also not inquisitive about why we are showing her hundreds of hours of faces. She is extremely passive and doesn't show any interest. She doesn't have a mechanism to tell her what is interesting to asking about in the world.

References

Anderson AK, Phelps EA 2000 Expression without recognition: contributions of the human amygdala to emotional communication. Psychol Sci 11:106–111

Hamada T, McLean WH, Ramsay M et al 2002 Lipoid proteinosis maps to 1q21 and is caused by mutations in the extracellular matrix protein 1 gene (ECM1). Hum Mol Genet 11:833–840

Smith ML, Cottrell GW, Gosselin F, Schyns PG 2005 Transmitting and decoding facial expressions. Psychol Sci 16:184–189

Models of distributive justice

Jonathan Wolff

Department of Philosophy, University College London, Gower Street, London WC1E 6BT, UK

Abstract. Philosophical disagreement about justice rages over at least two questions. The most immediate is a substantial question, concerning the conditions under which particular distributive arrangements can be said to be just or unjust. The second, deeper, question concerns the nature of justice itself. What is justice? Here we can distinguish three views. First, justice as mutual advantage sees justice as essentially a matter of the outcome of a bargain. There are times when two parties can both be better off by making some sort of agreement. Justice, on this view, concerns the distribution of the benefits and burdens of the agreement. Second, justice as reciprocity takes a different approach, looking not at bargaining but at the idea of a fair return or just price, attempting to capture the idea of justice as equal exchange. Finally justice as impartiality sees justice as 'taking the other person's point of view' asking 'how would you like it if it happened to you?' Each model has significantly different consequences for the question of when issues of justice arise and how they should be settled. It is interesting to consider whether any of these models of justice could regulate behaviour between non-human animals.

2006 Empathy and Fairness. Wiley, Chichester (Novartis Foundation Symposium 278) p 165–180

Questions of distributive justice arise, naturally enough, in contexts where some sort of goods or service could be provided for two or more people. The reason why this is of interest to philosophers is that in many cases disagreements are possible about what justice requires in a particular situation. There are also disagreements about how these disagreements are to be settled. These 'meta-disagreements' ultimately concern the nature of justice, as a philosophical concept, rather than disagreement over which are the 'correct' principles of justice. In this paper I shall consider the meta-debate: the philosophical question 'what is justice?'.

To anticipate, I am going to sketch out three competing accounts of justice, which can be called 'justice as mutual advantage'; 'justice as reciprocity' or fair exchange; and 'justice as impartiality', and I will illustrate some of the different implications of these accounts, and finally consider whether any of them can plausibly be applied to non-human animals. When philosophers have discussed these models, often they have taken their task to be to show which one is correct.[1] Here, though, my aim is to explain their differences and their presuppositions to see how this may illuminate issues concerning animal behaviour and capacities.

Like others, we can take as our starting point David Hume's influential conception of what is called 'the circumstances of justice' (Hume 1998). Hume argued that the concept of justice is not applicable to all situations in which issues of distribution are in question. There are, he says, both objective and subjective circumstances of justice. The objective circumstances concern the supply of the goods in question. If the goods were abundant, in the sense that everyone can have as much as they wish without reducing the quantity that others can take, issues of justice simply would not arise. Philosophers illustrate this with the example of manna from heaven, but under normal circumstances, air provides a good case. Given that there is so much air around no one need calculate how much others are using or complain that anyone is breathing too heavily. But this can change. Stuck in a lift, or trapped in a mine with the waters rising, we might think very differently. Yet under normal circumstances of abundance of air there is no need to complain if someone seems to be taking more than others, or 'wasting' it though unnecessarily vigorous exercise, for example. Some have argued that it is precisely because abundance takes us 'beyond justice' that Marx insisted that for communism to be possible it was necessary to achieve abundance (see, for example Lukes 1982).

At the other end of the scale, Hume argues that gross scarcity also makes justice inappropriate. This is more controversial, but Hume argues that if there is so little that people's survival is in doubt, no one can be criticized for taking and holding on to whatever they can. We could describe this as the view that there are circumstances where justice begins to become a luxury. But in sum, on Hume's view, justice is only relevant if the goods in question are neither grossly scarce or hugely abundant. These are the objective circumstances of justice. We need also pay attention to the subjective circumstances. Justice, Hume argues, only arises if there is the possibility of conflicts of interest. As Hume memorably puts it 'Why raise landmarks between my neighbour's field and mine, when my heart has made no division between our interests; but shares all his joys and sorrows with the same force and vivacity as if originally my own?'[2] On Hume's view sometimes some families approach this state and within such families ideas of justice are out of place. Finally, and this was famously disputed by Kant, Hume supposes that if someone were to fall among 'ruffians' who were so debased as to have no disposi-

---

[1] In fact, the distinction between these models has only recently been clarified, especially in work by Brian Barry, and so elements that properly belong in different models, at least according to this analysis, are sometimes joined together. I will ignore this complication here. (See Barry 1989, 1996, Buchanan 1990, Gibbard 1991, Wolff 1998.)

[2] Hume, op. cit.

tion to equity and order, at the least such a person could not be criticized for doing whatever could be done to preserve his own life (Kant 1991).

Although Hume's account of the circumstances of justice has been influential, Hume's own theory of the nature of justice brings out its consequences when understood as he intended. Essentially, Hume's central thesis is that ideas of justice only have a place where cooperation has a point for everyone involved in the situation. We can put this in terms of the idea of mutual advantage: if everyone went their separate ways, they would achieve a particular result. However with the cooperation of others, they can each do better. A surplus is possible. Justice then is a matter of working out rules for the division of the benefit provided by cooperation. We can see how this relates to the objective circumstances of justice. Where there is already abundance cooperation yields no benefits; where there is extreme scarcity, even after cooperation, then again it is pointless.

Although this may seem quite reasonable, it can generate the view that justice is a type of bargain, in which those with the greatest bargaining power will, as a matter of justice, receive most. Note that bargaining power is determined by how much one—or rather one's agreement—is needed by others, and not the extent of one's contribution. This we see, rather chillingly, illustrated in Hume's own application of his theory, worth quoting at length:

> Were there a species of creatures intermingled with men, which, though rational, were possessed of such inferior strength, both of body and mind, that they were incapable of all resistance, and could never, upon the highest provocation, make us feel the effects of their resentment; the necessary consequence, I think, is that we should be bound by the laws of humanity to give gentle usage to these creatures, but should not, properly speaking, lie under any restraint of justice with regard to them, nor could they possess any right or property, exclusive of such arbitrary lords. Our intercourse with them could not be called society, which supposes a degree of equality; but absolute command on the one side, and servile obedience on the other. Whatever we covet, they must instantly resign: Our permission is the only tenure, by which they hold their possessions: Our compassion and kindness the only check, by which they curb our lawless will: And as no inconvenience ever results from the exercise of a power, so firmly established in nature, the restraints of justice and property, being totally USELESS, would never have place in so unequal a confederacy.
>
> This is plainly the situation of men, with regard to animals; and how far these may be said to possess reason, I leave it to others to determine. The great superiority of civilized Europeans above barbarous Indians, tempted us to imagine ourselves on the same footing with regard to them, and made us throw off all restraints of justice, and even of humanity, in our treatment of them. In many nations, the female sex are reduced to like slavery, and are rendered incapable of all property, in opposition to their lordly masters. But though the males, when united, have in all countries bodily force sufficient to maintain this severe tyranny, yet such are the insinuation, address, and charms of their fair companions, that women are commonly able to break the confederacy, and share with the other sex in all the rights and privileges of society.[3]

---

[3] Hume op. cit.

The logic, then, of Hume's position is that if others have nothing to offer us, or things we can take from them independently of what they decide or want, then we have no duties of justice, strictly speaking, towards them. Hume does not deny that we have moral duties of humanity in such cases, but not of justice.

The obvious point to make in response is that this simply doesn't sound much like justice, in that it allows one person or group to take from another without making what would appear to be proper payment. Indeed justice as mutual advantage seems a very primitive idea of justice, in which 'might makes right'. The only reason for restraint, from the point of view of justice, is to try to establish a general atmosphere of co-operation, which will be in my long-term interests, rather than allow a damaging power struggle. Justice and long-term self-interest of the powerful seem to converge.

Unhappiness with the idea that 'proper payment' is missing from justice as mutual advantage generates the next theory of justice, which was called 'justice as reciprocity' above, but might be called 'justice as fair exchange'. On this view justice requires not so much bargaining as proportionality: those who make the greatest contribution should, in justice, receive the greatest return. It is easy to see that ideas of desert naturally fit into this picture, although as soon as this is said it will also be seen that there are many ways of fleshing this out. Does desert attach to effort? Or to achievement? Or to some hybrid of the two? Many theories are possible, but the general notion of justice as fair exchange has great resonance with many people, underlying slogans such as 'a fair day's pay for a fair day's work'. It is this notion which makes the biblical 'parable of the workers in the field' so troubling. In this story the farm-owner pays the same both to those who have worked only half a day and those who have worked a whole day. Although the farmer appeals to the argument that those who worked the full day received exactly what they were promised, it is very easy to see why they should have thought themselves hard-done by.

While justice as reciprocity appears intuitively more acceptable, a problem with both justice as mutual advantage and justice as reciprocity is that they leave out those who may have nothing to contribute or exchange. Consider those people who are so severely disabled that they are unable to make any productive contribution. Few will want to argue that such people are not owed anything by those who are able to work, but our question is whether these are duties of justice or, perhaps, merely of charity. On the two views discussed so far there is no obvious way of generating duties of justice. But to many this will seem wrong, and that others have a duty of justice to help the unfortunate. A different theory is needed to explain this.

The most prominent candidate is 'justice as impartiality', where justice requires taking everyone's situation and interests into account in determining what is to count as a just outcome. Here mechanisms for determining just outcomes take as their inspiration the thought 'how would you like it if you were in that situation?' So, for example, Adam Smith's device of the 'impartial spectator' (Smith 2002), or more recently John Rawls's 'veil of ignorance'(Rawls 1971) require the decision maker to take on the perspective of every individual involved or affected. To apply Rawls' model to the case of the disabled (something Rawls himself does not do, in fact) would be to ask the question: 'what provisions for the disabled would you want in your society if you didn't know whether or not you were disabled?' Here a balance needs to be struck between the interests of those who are disabled, and those who will have to work to provide things that the disabled cannot provide for themselves. Nevertheless, one may conjecture that if this method were seriously applied then arrangements for the disabled may be more congenial than they presently are, at least in some societies.

In considering whether behaviour between animals could be regulated by norms of justice that correspond to these models, we should note that each model is more demanding, both cognitively and morally than the previous one. Hence justice as mutual advantage is a fairly minimal standard, and requires a creature only, first, to be able to distinguish immediate interest from longer term interest, and second, to understand that other creatures may well modify their behaviour in the light of their expectation of how others will behave. In other words, it requires animals to be able to behave as game theorists, in a dynamic environment, rather than as decision theorists making choices in a static environment. It is not implausible that evolutionary mechanisms could encourage the development of such traits in some animals, and it would not be a surprise to learn that animals can develop forms of cooperation which yield outcomes that are consistent with justice as mutual advantage.

Justice as reciprocity or fair exchange requires a much more sophisticated understanding. Specifically it requires a creature to be able to deploy a concept of proportionality. This could be proportion between effort and reward for an individual, or, across individuals, an idea of similar treatment. In the latter context I understand that there is experimental evidence that some apes are able to make this judgement, refusing to accept a lesser 'payment' when another ape has been lavishly paid for undertaking the same task. Note, though, this does not seem to require empathy in the sense of seeing things from another's point of view. Rather it requires only some notion of comparison. Note, too, that a sense of *injustice* is not yet the same as a sense of *justice*. The latter would be displayed by the lucky ape offering a portion of the over-payment to the unlucky ape. Observing this would be very interesting indeed. It would be hard to see what could motivate such behaviour, if it were ever to happen, other than a sense of empathy.

The final idea of justice, justice as impartiality, also requires empathy. We should note, however, that this is not the empathy a mother may have for her offspring, which can be closer to a sense of merging identities, but rather empathy for another creature understood as a distinct individual. It would be consistent, for example, with a group of animals sharing their kill with a member of the group who is too old and infirm to perform any useful task, and yet is not a family member. However, even if such behaviour is observed no doubt there would be competing explanations, perhaps based on an 'accidental over-spill' of norms of mutual advantage.

In conclusion, in understanding whether animals are capable of following norms of justice, and the relation between justice and empathy, it is important to keep in mind that there are different models of justice, not all of which pre-suppose empathy. Hence one must be clear in each case which model of justice is in play, and what conceptual demands it makes on its participants. Keeping this in mind may help understand and classify animal capacities and forms of behaviour.

References

Barry B 1989 Theories of justice. University of California Press, Berkeley

Barry B 1996 Justice as impartiality. Oxford University Press, Oxford

Buchanan A 1990 Justice as reciprocity versus subject-centered justice. Philos Public Aff 19:227–252

Gibbard A 1991 Constructing justice. Philos Public Aff 20:264–279

Hume D 1998 An enquiry concerning the principles of morals section III Part 1. Oxford University Press, Oxford

Kant I 1991 Idea for a universal history [Idea for a universal history with a cosmopolitan purpose], in Reiss Kant, Political writings, trans. Nisbet HB (ed) with an introduction and notes by H. Reiss. Cambridge University Press, Cambridge, p 41–53

Lukes S 1982 Marxism, morality and justice. Parkinson GHR (ed) Marx and Marxism. Cambridge University Press, Cambridge, p 177–205

Rawls J 1971 A theory of justice. Oxford University Press, Oxford

Smith A 2002 Theory of the moral sentiments (ed) K Haakonssen. Cambridge University Press, Cambridge Part 3, Chapter 3

Wolff J 1998 Rational, fair and reasonable. In: Kelly P (ed) Impartiality, neutrality and justice: re-reading Brian Barry's Justice as impartiality. Edinburgh University Press, Edinburgh, p 35–43

DISCUSSION

Brosnan: I did the studies on reactions to inequity in non-human primates that you mentioned (Brosnan & de Waal 2004, Brosnan et al 2005). These were the studies done in both chimpanzees and capuchin monkeys in which two primates were paired and then performed a simple exchange task for food. One of the primates would sometimes get a better reward, a grape, while the other monkey got a cucumber. In both cases, the disadvantaged primate (the one who got the cucumber) reacted negatively to the inequity, often refusing to complete the exchange or accept the food reward. However, in neither species did the advantaged partner (the one getting the better grape) try to rectify the inequity by sharing with the disadvantaged partner. In the capuchins we saw no examples of sharing by the advantaged partner and in the chimpanzees, we saw only five instances out of 2000 trials. This is dramatically less than the normal rates of sharing in this group of chimpanzees, so if anything they were inhibiting their willingness to share. There have since been studies done by two groups in which chimpanzees were set up in a situation in which they could give their partner a reward at no cost to themselves, and they were indifferent to this possibility (Silk et al 2005, also see Jensen et al 2006). They weren't spiteful, but they weren't prosocial, either. It looks like we are seeing a situation with only disadvantageous inequity aversion. They don't like it when they get less than a conspecific partner, but they don't seem to care about their partner's well-being, either. In a further follow-up study I looked at their actions: in this they apparently pay attention to the actions of their partners, but as far as I can tell this is in terms of whether or not being nice will get them more in the long-run than not being nice will. I agree with you that it is justice by reciprocity at this point.

Wolff: It might not even be as much as justice by reciprocity. When I first heard about this work, I assumed they had made comparisons about how much work they had done to get the reward, but it sounds like now they are not even doing this.

Brosnan: There was an element of effort involved, too. We included a small effort component, which is the exchange I mentioned previously. We did see much stronger reactions when there was unequal effort in capuchins, indicating that they are paying attention to effort, but this was not the case with the chimpanzees.

Hauser: It is interesting to hear the comment about Hume, because Rawls, in the original position, never mentioned sex as one of the distinguishing things in his 'veiled ignorance' method. That is, if you want impartiality, he wanted to exclude things like age, education and race, but never invoked sex or gender as a biasing factor. You didn't mention Rawls' equation: for him, justice is fairness. His last book, a follow-up to the *Theory of Justice* is called *Justice as Fairness.* I bring this up because of the work that Frolich & Oppenheimer (1993) have done in political science, where they try to get people to either work out a set a of fair principles, or decide which of a set of suggested principles would be best, and then work through an artificial economic system that implements these principles. People don't necessarily come up with the Rawlsian principles explicitly; they aim at the idea that society should support the least advantaged while simultaneously rewarding effort. It goes beyond Rawls in that it does put in the effort, but it also takes advantage of his notion that you want some floor below which you never go. With these artificial conditions, set up for subjects in Poland, China, the USA and other countries, one finds relatively similar principles emerging. Does this have any value in terms of intuition?

Wolff: There are various types of social psychology studies asking what people think about distributive justice. One of the findings that is most robust is agreement with the principle that those who work harder should get more than those who don't work so hard. In one study, I think 96% strongly agreed or agreed. It would be nice to meet the 4% who didn't! From the perspective of political philosophy, the difficulty has always been to make this intuition into a normative theory. What does it mean to work harder? Is it to produce more, or to put in more effort? Typically we think that people who put in lots of effort but don't produce much should get the sack, but from the point of view of desert theory, maybe they are the ones that should be getting more? What are the proxies for working hard here? In Rawls' case part of the problem will be the desert base: the characteristics you have in virtue of which you can be deserving. This desert base may be partially undeserved. How can people who inherit a talent and can earn more be deserving of this? Yet in most areas of employment there is no resentment when the promotion goes to the person who is better at the job, whether they inherited that skill or not. We have intuitions about rewarding desert and rewarding undeserved talent which cut against the orthodoxy of much left-wing political philosophy.

Gergely: You said very little about the impartiality model. How does this differ from Marx's view that in a 'fair' society (of future communism) everyone should receive as much of the resources as they personally have a need for?

Wolff: That is a good question. For Hume, transcending justice requires a kind of dissolving of identity or personality between people. Typically, impartiality doesn't require this much, but it does seem to require something pretty strong. Some of those who have argued in favour of impartiality models, such as some of the utilitarians, had proposed that we should imagine an impartial spectator who takes on everyone's interests. Yet the impartiality model is meant to be a theory of justice, not a theory beyond justice. The only way I can make sense of this is to think of the Hume model as imagining impartiality on a day-to-day basis, so you live your life not distinguishing your interests from those of others, whereas in the impartiality model of justice, it is a type of theoretical reflection: what principles would we adopt if we didn't know what place we would play in society. This would lead to principles of a safety net: no one would do too badly. If we didn't know our place, we would make sure everyone was OK. Rawls says that if we were to think this through, our first thought would be that we should share everything out equally. But we know from human psychology that often people respond better to incentives. We can do much better if we allow some inequalities, which will then raise the position of the worst off. Even though this is an impartiality model of justice, it does allow that people will often act selfishly in their own lives. We have to set up a basic structure that recognizes we are humans with our own foibles. We need institutions and background structures to put the impartiality model in place.

Van Lange: I think that the taxonomy can be mapped on to situations. For example, the first one, a bargain one, is applicable to situations where there is a single interactions. The reciprocity based one can only be applied to repeated interactions. The last one, empathy based, has a lot of generality, but empathy is not always there. I wonder about justice in society, because reciprocity is not a good system for larger groups. What kind of system would apply at a societal level?

Wolff: These models of justice are not themselves meant to generate principles that apply directly to society. In terms of reciprocity, justice does not give us instructions to equalize every transaction. Rather, it gives a background understanding of what types of principles might be appropriate or not. A desert model would be an example of the reciprocity theory of justice. It tries to reward people on the basis of a fair foundation. Where societies don't seem to have any basis of reward according to desert, there seems to be a lack of affiliation: people become alienated from that society if they see no relation between hard work and reward. There is a notion of reciprocity that works there. One way of interpreting what you said is if you think of a game theoretic perspective: in the end, everything is self interest. If everything is self interest, then in a one-off interaction you get everything you can, but over a long term you need to understand about reputation and so on. In a face-to-face society where you know everyone and your reputation is clear, then morality and self-interest coincide. But in a modern society where we are alienated from each other and you can interact with many different people, then maybe bargaining comes back into it. You can model a lot of this in terms of game theory, but broadly this is not a popular move among political philosophers, on the grounds that they don't accept the starting premise of essential self interest in human behaviour.

C Frith: What I thought was interesting in the last, empathy based case is the implication that if you were unable to take a perspective other than your own, certain kinds of justice would not be visible to you. This would apply perhaps to people with autism.

U Frith: That is a valid point. According to this, you would readily perceive your own rights but nothing else.

Wolff: My knowledge of autism is what I read in the Sunday supplements, so I am not in a position to comment in detail. But from popular understanding I think that would be right. I think it would take you as far as the reciprocity model. It would allow comparisons, as long as they are all in the external world rather than the mind. Are people with autism able to tell how much effort other people are putting into things?

U Frith: It is difficult to answer that, but it is known that autistic people feel that they are owed things, and complain that people are nasty to them. There is an interesting, strong feeling of injustice but it is very self-centred.

Wolff: It is interesting, because you then have to ask, justice in virtue of what? Rights in virtue of what? What is the answer for this in the mind of the autistic person? Is it justice because I am a human being like every other human being?

U Frith: Yes. They are claiming, 'I have a rough deal. I have lots of difficulties.'

Wolff: We have this notion of being a moral agent. What is the other side of this? In a way, it is being a moral subject or patient, someone that morality applies to. It may well be that what you are describing is half of the impartiality picture, from the patient's point of view rather than the agent's point of view.

U Frith: I have just remembered that there is one bit of bargaining element that is prominent in discussions among autistics. They like to claim that many famous people through history have had autism and have been of immense value to society.

Wolff: Again, the return for reward is present, in that their contribution to society needs to be recognized and rewarded.

Frank: Has the moral philosophy community taken account of this shift in the link between effort or talent and reward? There has recently been an explosion of the difference in what you get as a function of very small differences in what you do. Everyone wanted to hear the best tenor in 1900, as they do now. We needed 10 000 tenors then; now three tenors can record all the recordings that people want to listen to. If you are just a little better than the next best you get paid seven figures, while the rest teach middle-school students to sing in choruses for very little. Yet people seem to have this sense that they are entitled to their pre-tax income if that is what the market decided that they are worth. But there doesn't seem to be a discussion about why someone 1/1000 better than someone else gets 10 000 times more.

Wolff: Partly, most philosophers would say it is so obviously wrong that there is little more to discuss. Brian Barry published a book recently called *Why Social Justice Matters* (Barry 2005). It is a polemical book, pointing out that the economic models are very clear about why there should be such extremes. Barry argues that they have no foundation in justice. However there is some intuitive line of argument. The modern version of a bargaining morality is that the market tells us what justice is. If people are willing to pay for this, who are we to argue? This goes along with the idea that crtitics are trying to impose their values on the democratic market. There is a popularist libertarian view that the market tells us what everything is worth, and anyone who suggests an alternative is being autocratic. Most political philosophers haven't engaged in this sort of argument. There will have to be discussion of this because it is not something that is going away.

C Frith: There is beginning to be a little bit of punishment. Wasn't there a story about a famous German violinist whose fee became so great that one of the London orchestras refused to hire him?

Wolff: There has been an attempt to rein it in.

Hauser: There was also an incredible outcry against a guy from the New York stock exchange.

Frank: Occasionally these salaries aren't merited, but the main reason those salaries are so big is that if you make one or two decisions a little bit better with a $15 billion enterprise, the bottom line difference is way more than they are paying you. In terms of the value of your good decision, it is incredibly high.

Gallese: I am naïve and ignorant in this field, but I was thinking about the relationship between the notion of fairness and the notion of distributive justice. Are we entitled to the intuition that one single theory of distributive justice might be fair in all domains of application? I am considering how I may react to a decision taken by my government with respect to my father, dealing with the distribution of goods. My subjective reaction could be very different because my personal relationship as a patient with the agent of the enforcement of such justice reliant on a given model could be different.

Wolff: I have a couple of responses. One concerns a question that I didn't answer earlier, which was why did Rawls call his theory justice as fairness? I didn't mention this because I don't find the idea of fairness any clearer than the idea of justice. I don't think we have a clear notion of what fairness requires, so you could have the same debate about the taxonomy of the theories of fairness. I don't think we get any conceptual clarification by thinking of justice in terms of fairness. In terms of a universal domain, political philosophers see a number of theories, and normally get into a dispute about which is correct. They come out of a seminar room disagreeing, but this doesn't matter because they don't have to do anything about it, other than come back and discuss it again. My view is that when intelligent people have gone to a lot of trouble to design a model, they probably have some part of the truth there. Rather than think these are competitive theories, it might be better to think of them as theories that govern different domains. When I first started thinking of this I was asked to give a paper on the principles of justice in the European Union (EU). I had as my starting point that justice is relative to cooperation, so we have to think of what form of cooperation the EU is. At one end it could be a group of nations huddling together for strength, as a mutual protection agency, where a bargaining model of justice might be appropriate between them. But if you read the preamble to the various treaties they talk about ever-closer union, as if we are aiming at some complete submersion of interests. In this case it would look more like an impartiality model. Once we have ascertained the type of situation we are in we can begin to think of the type of norm that applies to this situation. Perhaps international relations is one where the bargaining model can apply, although in many cases we are beyond that and into reciprocity. If you think about international distributive justice, the idea that we should have it across borders, this has no prospect of success. It is not an appealing model to anyone, perhaps because we don't think we are part of that community. But we are a member of another type of community where we shouldn't be doing harm to each other.

Gallese: So universality is not at stake.

Wolff: It comes and goes as an issue. When Rawls was writing in 1971, it wasn't an issue. Everyone assumed he was writing a theory of justice that was valid for all times and all places. He never said this, but he was criticised on the grounds that his theory only seemed suitable for western democracies. He then said this is what he meant. A peculiar thing about political philosophy is that there is a huge amount of interest in people asserting things about universal human rights, but almost none of this is coming from philosophers, who are now thinking in more contextual terms.

Singer: I have a question about the impartiality model. You said that this model is similar to the empathy model. With regard of how we define empathy, as the ability to put oneself in someone else's shoes, I question however, if empathy is really necessary for an impartiality model? Is this model not based on what we would call an allocentric view, which is the capacity for abstract reasoning in the sense of taking into account all the different needs, including those of others? You would probably need high reasoning and cognitive perspective abilities for that.

Wolff: I am conscious from this meeting that you are making more distinctions among yourselves than moral philosophers would about empathy. Perhaps what you mean by empathy isn't the notion of empathy behind the model I described. All that is needed to get Rawls' model going is the ability to think 'how would I like to live in a society where I had no talents or in a group that is currently discriminated against'. Perhaps the only way to imagine this would be to think about people who are like this in real life, but this may not be necessary. The power of the Rawlsian approach is that most of us don't think of what it would be like to live in a society if you were very different from how you are. If you had an IQ of 80 and you left school when you were 15, would this be a good society to live in? His methodology is to think how we can make society a good place to live in for someone like that. Does it require empathy to answer that question?

Singer: I would say yes, but I could imagine arguments against that.

Wolff: What Rawls does is that he uses the device of ignorance as a way of modelling impartiality here. It is a model of impartiality, rather than empathy. He can reduce the situation to letting one person choose the principles for the whole of society. This person doesn't know their race, intelligence or sex. The brilliance of this is that ignorance forces you to think in an impartial way. People have tried to do it the other way round with full knowledge models, but they are much more complicated and it is difficult to get anything determinant out of them.

Singer: When you say 'ignorance', you may be ignorant about your own future, but you need a lot of information on others' states to know how it would be to be them.

Wolff: You need knowledge about the general laws of psychology, economics and social science. You need to know also that your society is not in grave scarcity or huge abundance. He uses the Humeian idea that you have to know your society is within the circumstances of justice and that people have a conception of the good, and are capable of a sense of justice.

Hauser: One other thing that goes along with this is the notion of considered judgement, where Rawls states that you need to disregard emotions in working through the principles. An interesting historical note is that embedded in a footnote at the end of *A theory of justice* is a discussion he had with Robert Trivers, who produced a paper on reciprocal altruism (Trivers 1971) in the same year as the book. As a graduate student I had long conversations about Trivers' paper, which is where Rawls' inspiration about sociobiological theories of selfishness were triggered. Trivers tells me that Rawls' initial views were less well informed about the nature of selfish human nature. In some sense, Rawls' unique perspective is due to his appreciation of human selfishness, and the need to engage this while keeping everyone under a veil of ignorance to achieve impartiality. It is his unique contribution to the tradition of philosophers who used a social contract model.

Frank: The way that I understood that Rawls' exercise is that he wanted me, the reader, to agree that fairness required that we give a lot of attention to the people at the bottom of the queue, just out of fear that we might occupy a position like that. I am meant to be thinking about my risk of ending up in that position, and the fear of that outcome makes me grudgingly concede that fairness requires that we have to do a lot for that person. But the rules don't get passed behind a veil of ignorance. Rawls didn't want to use empathy or concern about other people to get us to admit fairness requires that we try to promote the welfare of those at the bottom; we make the rules knowing well who has what talents. How do you get people, once they are out from behind the veil of ignorance, to give due concern to the people at the bottom? There you need to encourage people to call on what resources of empathy they might be able to draw on.

C Frith: You seem to be saying that in order to develop these rules you have to eliminate emotion. One of the themes of our earlier discussions was that emotions help you to make good decisions. This would apply especially when you are making social decisions. There is a sort of intuitive or automatic sense of fairness and justice that we have, but can't really explain. To some extent what law is about is whether there is some way of codifying this intuitive sense of fairness that we have. You can see law as a constant attempt to produce written down rules that everyone will agree are just. This doesn't usually work so there is a constant mismatch between natural justice and the law. How does this relationship work, and where does the intuitive sense of fairness and justice come from.

Hauser: Your comments make a perfect link with Rawls. When Rawls suggested the linguistic analogy he was thinking of the operative principles as opposed to those that are expressed, or deployed in actual behaviour. There was an interesting book called *Fairness Versus Welfare* by Kaplow & Shavell (2002), two economists and legal scholars who approached the American legal system from the perspective of individual welfare. If you take this perspective, individuals would actually do quite a bit better in terms of various measures of utility than current fairness-based policy. They point out that we have such a reflexive response to thinking about the world in terms of fairness that we are virtually incapable of seeing the virtue of policy that runs counter to fairness, but leads to higher utility per individual. This is where the intuitive biases come into conflict with the proscriptive distinctions. What I would advocate is a legal system that is deeply sensitive to human nature, but never buying its intuitive judgments.

Montague: We have a long history in the USA of making proscriptions as egalitarian as possible, and not crafting them to individual welfare. If you are marginalized by the fact that you have an IQ of 80 and grew up in a low SES environment, it isn't acceptable in the USA to propose a situation that is good for you. We have this flawed notion that someone ought to have the same distribution of opportunity at the beginning of the game. Yet biology cripples that argument from the onset. People don't start out equal, but we pretend we can ignore this and the rules then get goofy when we try to patch things up retrospectively.

Blair: The trouble with the legal system is that it is largely influenced by the people in power. The people in power aren't particularly motivated to give maximum welfare to other individuals. One of the biggest mismatches is between what people do feel and what the ruling class wants them to feel, or wants to have instantiated to control the masses. You can't disentangle these huge sociological issues from this discussion.

Wolff: I haven't read the Kaplow and Shavell book, but I have heard of it. It is well known that if you have any type of view of fairness or moral privilege, this will lead to suboptimal outcomes in welfare terms. Their work is reminding us of something that has been known for a long time. There are discussions about this in moral philosophy in terms of partiality, that is, the right to be partial. A lot of people mention Dickens' Mrs Jellyby, who neglects her children in order to feed the starving children of Africa. This is the welfare-enhancing policy, yet we think of it as inhuman for her to do it. Much of our individual life is a matter of building relationships with other people and caring for them in this individual way. It may be true that we would maximize welfare in society if we ignored the attachment to our own children and gave our money to others, but this would go against what we think is the stuff of human life. This has to be part of the evolutionary discussion here about what is possible. It is distinct from anything to do with laws.

Montague: We would think of this as a welfare-disenhancing policy because of the need of children for attachment.

Wolff: You can always come up with examples where welfare is maximized by doing things that are considered to be unacceptable.

Montague: There will always be a bit of ignorance: no matter how perfect you think a programme is there is a bit of ignorance where you got things wrong.

Van Lange: There are biases, too. Ask two people in a relationship how much they share in household tasks, and the two percentages added together will likely exceed 100. There may also be a bias in achievement: people overestimate their own achievement and merit. There is a pervasive bias in merit-based systems, especially when the criteria are more ambiguous.

Montague: It is clear that the science is still embryonic in terms of its capacity to inform policy on a society wide scale.

U Frith: Could you comment on the difference between the way we judge acts of commission and acts of omission? There could be some sort of biological bias here. Would these theories treat these symmetrically?

Wolff: These theories of justice don't have a particular bearing on this, but it is a major question in moral philosophy. There is nothing like a consensus on it. Within the utilitarian tradition there is no moral distinction here. This is often treated as an objection to utilitarianism because it has the consequence that you are as responsible for your omissions as your commissions. There are a few cases where an omission is just as bad as a commission. If you were sitting by a pool next to a drowning child and you did nothing to save them even though this would have been easy to do, this would be seen to be almost as bad as pushing the child in. But I don't think there is a good philosophical argument for why there should be these intuitively held difference.

C Frith: The work Patrick Haggard has been doing about action and agency may be relevant here. The brain does a process called intentional binding, where it pulls together various acts such as pressing a button and a light coming on. There seems to be a built in mechanism that relates actions to their consequence (Haggard et al 2002). Presumably there is no such mechanism that can relate non-actions to their consequences.

Hauser: It is much more complicated than that. It is not just that we always have an action/omission bias: there are cases where we do not. What are the psychological parameters that trigger a strong action/omission bias and which do not?

Wolff: One of the complicating factors is that for public policy reasons we have to make some distinctions. In this country there is no law that requires you to give emergency aid, so you wouldn't be prosecuted in the swimming pool case unless you had a special position of responsibility. Public policy needs cruder distinctions than we would want in moral philosophy. Yet when we are now doing moral philosophy a lot of our intuitions are attempts to justify things which are public policy doctrines. We are using public policy to drive intuitions for which there might never be a philosophical justification because they were only ever pragmatically adopted in the first place. This is a further complicating factor. We are not going to find a beautiful set of principles that generate exactly the public policy we have.

References

Barry B 2005 Why social justice matters. Polity, Oxford
Brosnan SF, de Waal FBM 2004 Reply to 'Inequity aversion in capuchins'. Nature 428:140
Brosnan SF, Schiff HC, de Waal FBM 2005 Tolerance for inequity may increase with social closeness in chimpanzees. Proc Roy Soc Lond Ser B 272:253–258
Haggard P, Clark S, Kalogeras J 2002 Voluntary action and conscious awareness. Nat Neurosci 5:382–385
Jensen K, Hare B, Call J, Tomasello M 2006 What's in it for me? Self-regard precludes altruism and spite in chimpanzees. Proc Roy Soc Lond Ser B 273:1013–1021
Kaplow L, Shavell S 2002 Fairness versus Welfare. Harvard University Press, Cambridge
Frohlich N, Oppenheimer JA 1993 Choosing justice: an experimental approach to ethical theory. University of California Press, Berkeley
Silk JB, Brosnan SF, Vonk J et al 2005 Chimpanzees are indifferent to the welfare of unrelated group members. Nature 437:1357–1359
Trivers RL 1971 The evolution of reciprocal altruism. Quart Rev Biol 46:35–57

When do we empathize?

Frédérique de Vignemont

Institute of Cognitive Science, 67 bd Pinel, 69675 Bron cedex, France

Abstract. According to a motor theory of empathy, empathy results from the automatic activation of emotion triggered by the observation of someone else's emotion. It has been found that the subjective experience of emotions and the observation of someone else experiencing the same emotion activate overlapping brain areas. These shared representations of emotions (SRE) could be the key for the understanding of empathy. However, if the automatic activation of SRE suffices to induce empathy, we would be in a permanent emotional turmoil. In contrast, it seems intuitively that we do not empathize all the time and that far from being automatic, empathy should be explained by a complex set of cognitive and motivational factors. I will provide here a new account of the automaticity of empathy, starting from a very simple question: when do we empathize? We need to distinguish clearly the activation of SRE and empathy. I will provide a model that accounts both for the automaticity of the activation of SRE and for the selectiveness of empathy. As Prinz (2002) says about imitation, the problem is not so much to account for the ubiquitous occurrence of empathy, but rather for its notorious non-occurrence in many situations.

2006 Empathy and Fairness. Wiley, Chichester (Novartis Foundation Symposium 278) p 181–196

According to a traditional view of the mind, we only have an indirect access to what the other thinks or feels through observation and inference. The discovery of mirror neurons in monkeys activated both during action observation and action execution has challenged this view and opened a new pathway for the understanding of intersubjectivity. All we need to do is to exploit one's own resources in order to simulate or recreate someone else's mental states in oneself from a first-person perspective. Functional brain imagery has been recently seeking evidence of overlapping brain activations between feeling and observing the same emotion. Until now, the neural basis of the following emotions and bodily sensations has been shown to be shared: disgust, fear, anger, sadness, happiness, pain, touch (e.g. Calder et al 2000, Carr et al 2003, George et al 1996, Gur et al 2002, Jackson et al 2005, Kesler-West et al 2001, Keyser et al 2004, Phillips et al 1998, Singer 2006, Wicker at al 2003).

Feeling an emotion and observing someone else displaying the same emotion activate the same cortical representation. These shared representations of emotions (SRE) could be the key to the understanding of empathy. We share the same emotion with someone else because the observation of her emotion triggers automatically the activation of the representation of this emotion from a first-person perspective. However, if the automatic activation of SRE sufficed to induce empathy, we would be in a permanent emotional turmoil. In contrast, it seems intuitively that we do not empathize all the time and that far from being automatic, empathy should be explained by a complex set of factors. I will here provide a new account of the automaticity of empathy, starting from a very simple question: when do we empathize?

The automaticity of empathy

A colleague feels deeply jealous of me because the head of the department decided to send me to a conference that he wanted to attend. Do I share his feeling of jealousy? How could I feel jealous of myself? I do not empathize with him even if I may understand his reaction and feel sorry for him. However, this seems incompatible with recent experimental results about emotions. Brain areas dedicated to subjective experiences of emotions and bodily sensations are activated when observing someone else experiencing the same emotion or sensations whatever the kind of stimulus that is used. It does not seem to matter whether subjects see an isolated body part being injured (Jackson et al 2005) or a facial expression of an unknown person (Adolphs 2002). It does not make a difference whether the study emphasizes the context inducing the sensation (Botvinick et al 2005) or the specific body location injured (Avenanti et al 2005). In all cases, the authors found shared representations of emotions and sensations that are automatically activated. By automatic, I mean that the activation of SRE is (1) systematic, (2) independent from the context and (3) without the need for any further triggering condition. These results argue in the direction of a bottom-up theory of empathy: a small amount of information of low level is sufficient to induce an empathetic activation, which would be automatic. As Preston & de Waal (2002, p 4) say:

> 'attended perception of the object's state automatically activates the subject's representations of the state, situation and object, and that activation of these representations automatically primes or generates the associated autonomic and somatic responses, unless inhibited.'

We may better understand their claim, shared by many in the neuroscience of empathy, if we come back to action observation and imitation. From the very beginning, the notion of empathy has been linked to actions. Theodor Lipps suggested that by internally imitating a facial expression, we have direct access to the emotion that trigger this facial expression. The existence of mirror matching systems was considered as a neural evidence of Lipp's theory. Gallese (2001), one of the leaders of this view, defends what he calls the 'shared manifold' hypothesis.

He claims that empathy and mirror neurons are just two different levels of description of the same phenomenon of intersubjectivity. Action representations are automatically activated during action observation, even if the movement is not performed by conspecifics (e.g. monkey, human or dogs), as long as it belongs to the motor repertoire of the observer (Buccino et al 2004). The perception of someone else moving suffices to elicit the mental simulation of the performed movement. Unless inhibited, this motor simulation does not remain off line and is physically executed. Imitation is a prepotent response tendency. Indeed, subjects make more errors and are slower to perform a movement when they watch an incongruent movement (e.g. they move their index finger while seeing the little finger moving) (Brass et al 2000). Even if movements observation interferes with action execution, still most of the time we do not imitate other people. Imitation is thus automatic, even if most of the time inhibited. One may then suggest that empathy is not different from imitation. They depend both on shared representations between self and other. They are both automatic. They both remain offline if inhibited. Consequently, several authors have provided what they call 'a motor theory of empathy'.

We have to distinguish between two interpretations of the motor theory of empathy. According to a strong version, you recognize the emotion of others through motor imitation (Gallese 2001, Carr et al 2003, Leslie et al 2004). Empathy is automatic because motor imitation is automatic. According to a weaker version, action should be viewed just as a model of understanding. Both actions and emotions involve representations shared between self and others. They obey the same kind of principles. However, it does not mean that empathy is motoric, even if empathy may share many features with imitation (Preston & de Waal 2002, de Vignemont 2004).

I will not argue here pro or against any of these versions of the motor theory of empathy. I will rather analyse one of the claims that they both make about the automaticity of empathy.

The limits of the motor theory of empathy

How far can we draw the parallel between empathy and imitation? There are at least four main differences. First, it seems that we cannot help but share someone else's sadness. In contrast, we imitate because we want to, in order to learn for instance. Second, empathy has a salient phenomenological dimension. I empathize with you if I subjectively experience the same emotion as you. Goldman (1995) describes it as an 'online simulation'. It is difficult to make sense of what empathy would be if it remains offline. In contrast, the study of motor imagery has provided evidence of offline imitation. Third, autism and psychopathy are sometimes described as deficits of empathy, but as far as I know, there is no pathological case of the reverse, that is, patients that would compulsively empathize all the time with everybody. In contrast, some patients with frontal lesion are no longer able to inhibit their motor simulation and compulsively imitate others (Luria 1966, Lhermitte 1986, Brass et al 2003). Fourth, many factors influence when we feel empathy. For instance, we empathize more with people we feel close to or people we think are fair, as shown by Singer (2006, this volume). In contrast, we may imitate everybody.

Let me pursue further on this latter feature of empathy. At the beginning, we saw that it is difficult to empathize with a subject-directed emotion (e.g. jealousy or angriness toward the empathizer). There are other cases that raise difficulties regarding the automaticity of empathy and that show the complexity of the factors influencing when we feel empathy. Imagine that you witness a mother very upset with her son Peter because he made a silly joke about his younger brother Jack who could have been hurt. There are several scenarios of how Peter may react. (a) He regrets what he did and cries. (b) He does not feel sorry, Jack deserved what he got and nothing bad really happened anyway. (c) He does not regret because he did not do anything. His mother is mistaken and he feels her reaction as unfair. With whom do you empathize? Intuitively, in (b) we feel empathy with the mother. In contrast in (c), we empathize with Peter and we feel his mother's behaviour unfair. In (a), the situation is more ambiguous. On the one hand, we may empathize with Peter, the crying little boy. On the other hand, we may empathize with the worried mother.

If we assume that empathy is automatic, then we would have to empathize with two contradictory emotions in all the scenarios, a consequence that goes against our intuition. One could then reply that the activation of one of the emotions inhibits the activation of the other. Then the question is why this emotion rather than that one. Do we choose with whom we empathize? It does not seem so. The fact that I challenge the automaticity of empathy does not imply that empathy is a voluntary process. We suggest only that empathy is not systematic and needs further additional factors to take place. Preston & de Waal (2002) acknowledge that different factors influence when we empathize, like the familiarity effect. Interestingly, all the factors they describe explain why we feel empathy in some cases, rather than why we do not feel empathy most of the time. Most of the literature about empathy has focused on the conditions that trigger empathy. However, if the activation of SRE sufficed to automatically induce empathy, then there would be no need for any further necessary conditions to explain why and when we feel empathy. As Prinz (2002) says about imitation, the problem is not so much to account for the ubiquitous occurrence of empathy, but rather for its notorious non-occurrence in many situations. The automatic activation of shared representations of emotions cannot be the whole story about empathy.

A two-step model

I would like to suggest here that the problem arises from a confusion in the litera-ture between empathy (sharing the emotional feeling) and SRE (sharing the corti-cal representation of the emotion). I will now try to provide a model that accounts both for the automaticity of the activation of SRE and for the selectiveness of empathy.

SRE and empathy

Interestingly, a shift in the studies about emotions happened recently. A number of studies have investigated how we recognize the emotions in others based on facial expressions without appealing to our own feelings: subjects have merely to categorize without experiencing the displayed emotion. Indeed, when I watch a face showing fear, I do not feel afraid. There is no empathy involved here. None-theless, brain imagery show activation of SRE. In contrast, recent studies on pain have emphasized the subjective phenomenology experienced by subjects while watching the others. When I watch someone being hurt by a needle, I feel almost as if that was happening to me. There is a salient phenomenological dimension of the first-person perspective. In this sense, there is empathy.

As Wicker et al (2003) notice, the strong version of the motor theory of empathy leads to a 'cold hypothesis', which merely requires sharing the facial motor repre-sentation of the emotion, in contrast with the 'hot hypothesis' that actually requires sharing the conscious feeling of the emotion. These two views of emotion recogni-tion should not be confused, nor should we reduce empathy to the mere activation of SRE. By definition, empathy involves the subject's emotional experiences and we need to take into account this phenomenological dimension.

We need to draw a sharp distinction between different levels of sharing of emo-tions. At a primary level, the observation of someone else's emotion triggers the activation of SRE. This activation is automatic and is not inhibited. It occurs independently of the context. It underlies the recognition of the emotion displayed. But the activation of SRE does not necessarily lead to the phenomenological expe-rience of the emotion and can remain offline. At a secondary level, one has con-scious access to the emotion associated with the activation of SRE. It is only then that one experiences the emotion of other. It is only then that we can talk of empathy. Far from being automatic, empathy depends on several contextual factors. Consequently, empathy does not need to be inhibited all the time, it is rather sometimes triggered by external conditions. The default rule is not that we empa-thize with everybody.

I will now turn on the different factors that mediate the transition between the primary and the secondary level, between SRE and empathy. I would like to suggest that there are at least two main mechanisms that are involved: the distinction between self and other and the evaluation of the emotional event.

Distinction between self and others

By definition, SRE encode both one's own emotions and emotions of others. They do not specify whose emotions they represent, mine or yours. SRE are intersubjective. The activation of SRE expresses this primary lack of differentiation between self and others. The lack of differentiation implies the necessity of disambiguating the representations by articulating who the subject is (de Vignemont 2004, Decety & Jackson 2004).

In this sense, shared representations of emotions are similar to shared representations of actions and we can go further in the parallel between emotion and action. The activation of mirror neurons does not suffice by itself to determine who is moving, because their content does not specify the agent. This is why we need an additional mechanism that enables us to self-attribute our own actions: the 'Who' system (de Vignemont & Fourneret 2004). Interestingly, this mechanism is also involved in the inhibition of imitation (Brass et al 2005). In contrast with other inhibition mechanisms that are involved for instance in the Stroop task, the inhibition of imitation activates the anterior fronto-median cortex and the temporal-parietal junction, which are both known to be involved in the sense of agency and in perspective-taking. Brass and colleagues claim that the distinction between internally generated and externally triggered motor representations plays a key role to prevent us to imitate someone else's movements. Put it another way, I do not imitate your movements because they are yours and they do not match my own intentions.

Similarly, I would like to suggest that I do not empathize with your emotions because they are yours and they do not match my global feelings and my emotional situation. A crucial requirement for the conscious experience of the emotion would thus be the distinction between my emotions and your emotions. If one detects that SRE are activated following the observation of someone else's emotion, then the activation of SRE does not lead to the phenomenological experience of the emotion in oneself. Indeed, why should one feel what the others feel? One can recognize the emotions of others based on SRE without having to experience them. The offline simulation of emotions suffices, there is no need for empathy. In contrast, if SRE are activated following the experience of an emotional event for oneself, then the activation of SRE leads to the phenomenological experience of the emotion in oneself. The distinction between self and others thus makes the difference between emotional experience in oneself and emotion recognition in others.

If this is true, then we would never empathize. However, we do empathize even when we do not necessarily want to. We need a further step to explain why we feel

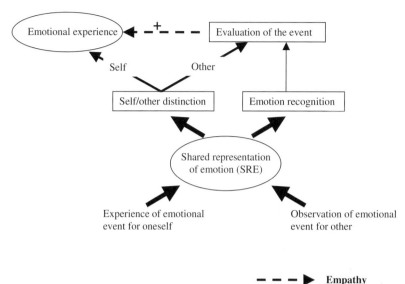

FIG. 1.   A two-step model of empathy.

someone else's emotions despite the fact that they are not our own emotions (see Fig. 1).

A set of complex factors

The hypothesis is that SRE are automatically activated in any emotional context, whether one is at the core of this context or someone else. If the subject of the emotion is the self, then the activation leads to an emotional experience. If the subject of the emotion is someone else, then there is no such experience, unless if other factors reinforce the activation of the SRE leading then to an emotional experience despite the fact that it's someone else's emotion. In this latter case, there is empathy. I would like now to review some of these factors that counterbalance the inhibition of SRE (see Table 1).

The evaluation of the emotional event is not performed voluntarily and remains implicit. The evaluation focuses on three poles: the emotion itself, the person who experiences the emotion and the empathizer.

The first main factor concerns the emotion that one shares with the other. We need again to distinguish between different dimensions. First, some emotions are easier to share than others, like for instance, sadness or pain. I would like to suggest that basic emotions are easier than complex ones and negative easier than positive. I also mentioned at the beginning the impossibility of empathizing for an emotion

TABLE 1   Main factors influencing when we empathize

Type of emotion	*Person feeling the emotion*	*Empathizer*
Target of the emotion	Familiarity	Gender
Complexity	Attitude toward the person	Level of attention
Valence	Similarity and identification	Emotional context
Emotional repertoire		
Saliency and intensity		
Justification		

directed toward the empathizer, like jealousy. Second, the shared emotion has to belong to one's own emotional repertoire (also called the effect of past experience by Preston and de Waal). If you don't suffer from vertigo, you can hardly empathize with me when I am frightened by the void below me. Similarly, the role of motor familiarity for mirror neurons has been demonstrated (Calvo-Merino et al 2005). Third, the shared emotion has to be salient. One does not feel empathy for weak emotions, but rather for strong ones that capture our attention. Four, the shared emotion has to be consistent with the internal and external background. According to a simulationist approach, we put ourselves in someone else's shoes based on the simulation of the mental states of the person and of the context. For instance, can we empathize with someone who starts suddenly screaming and crying with no obvious reason? I predict that we would be surprised rather than share her state of distress. In our previous example, when the mother is unfair with Peter (c), it is difficult to share her anger because we know it is not justified.

The relationship between the empathizer and the subject is also important. This relationship can be understood in three ways. First, there is the familiarity effect as described by Preston & de Waal (2002): we empathize more with relatives or people that we know well. That could be easily explained if we assume a simulation- ist approach: the more we know about the other, the easier it gets to put oneself in their shoes. Second, there is the emotional attitude that the empathizer has for the subject. That's what Tania Singer shows in her study: men empathize less with people they think unfair (see this volume). Third, there is the similarity effect, also pointed out by Preston and de Waal. We empathize more with people we can iden- tify to. Then I can really feel the same emotion as if I were you. The dimmer the boundary between the self and other, the easier it is to go beyond this boundary.

A third factor is the overall personal context of the empathizer. According to Baron-Cohen & Wheelwright (2004), women have a higher empathy score than men. More importantly, we are not open to others all the time, paying attention to what they feel. When all our needs are satisfied, we are more likely to empathize (Hoffman 1975). For instance, happy children empathize more (Strayer 1980).

Other factors may also play a role and need to be experimentally investigated. Furthermore, each factor may provide a contradictory response and will have to be pondered differently. That will decide in the end whether we feel empathy or not.

Conclusion

The discovery of SRE has opened up a new pathway for the understanding of empathy but does not suffice in itself as a full account of the complexity of when we empathize. I suggested here that we should distinguish between SRE and empathy. While SRE remains offline, empathy is characterized by the phenomeno-logical experience of someone else's emotion. While the activation of SRE is automatic, empathy is selective. Further work needs to be done to understand the transition from one to the other.

References

Adolphs R 2002 Neural systems for recognizing emotion. Curr Opinion Neurobiol 12: 169–177

Avenanti A, Bueti D, Galati G, Aglioti SM 2005 Transcranial magnetic stimulation highlights the sensorimotor side of empathy for pain. Nat Neurosci 8:955–960

Baron-Cohen S, Wheelwright S 2004 The empathy quotient: an investigation of adults with Asperger syndrome or high functioning autism and normal sex differences. J Autism Dev Disord 34:163–175

Botvinick M, Jha AP, Bylsma LM, Fabian SA, Solomon PE, Prkachin KM 2005 Viewing facial expressions of pain engages cortical areas involved in the direct experience of pain. Neuroim-age 25:312–319

Brass M, Bekkering H, Wohlschlager A, Prinz W 2000 Compatibility between observed and executed finger movements: comparing symbolic, spatial, and imitative cues. Brain Cogn 44:124–143

Brass M, Derrfuss J, Matthes-von Cramon G, von Cramon DY 2003 Imitative response tenden-cies in patients with frontal brain lesions. Neuropsychology 17:265–271

Brass M, Derrfuss J, von Cramon DY 2005 The inhibition of imitative and overlearned responses: a functional double dissociation. Neuropsychologia 43:89–98

Buccino G, Lui F, Canessa N et al 2004 Neural circuits involved in the recognition of actions performed by nonconspecifics: an FMRI study. J Cogn Neurosci 16:114–126

Calder AJ, Keane J, Manes F, Antoun N, Young AW 2000 Impaired recognition and experience of disgust following brain injury. Nat Neurosci 3:1077–1078

Calvo-Merino B, Glaser DE, Grezes J, Passingham RE, Haggard P 2005 Action observation and acquired motor skills: an FMRI study with expert dancers. Cereb Cortex 15:1243–1249

Carr L, Iacoboni M, Dubeau MC, Mazziotta JC, Lenzi GL 2003 Neural mechanisms of empathy in humans: a relay from neural systems for imitation to limbic areas. Proc Natl Acad Sci USA 100:5497–5502

de Vignemont F 2004 The co-consciousness hypothesis: from mirror neurons to empathy. Phenomenology and Cognitive Sciences 13:97–114

de Vignemont F, Fourneret P 2004 The sense of agency: a philosophical and empirical review of the 'Who' system. Conscious Cogn 13:1–19

Decety J, Jackson PL 2004 The functional architecture of human empathy. Behav Cogn Neurosci Rev 3:71–100

Gallese V 2001 The 'shared manifold' hypothesis: from mirror neurons to empathy. Journal of Consciousness Studies 8:33–50

George MS, Ketter TA, Parekh PI, Herscovitch P, Post RM 1996 Gender differences in regional cerebral blood flow during transient self-induced sadness or happiness. Biol Psychiatry 40:859–871

Goldman A 1995 Empathy, mind and morals. In: Davies M & Stone S (eds) Mental simulation: Philosophical and psychological essays. Blackwells, Oxford, p 185–208

Gur RC, Schroeder L, Turner T et al 2002 Brain activation during facial emotion processing. NeuroImage 16:651–662

Hoffman ML 1975 Developmental synthesis of affect and cognition and its implication for altruistic motivation. Dev Psychobiol 11:607–622

Jackson PL, Meltzoff AN, Decety J 2005 How do we perceive the pain of others? A window into the neural processes involved in empathy. NeuroImage 24:771–779

Kesler-West ML, Andersen AH, Smith CD et al 2001 Neural substrates of facial emotion processing using fMRI. Cogn Brain Res 11:213–226

Keysers C, Wicker B, Gazzola V, Anton JL, Fogassi L, Gallese V 2004 A touching sight: SII/PV activation during the observation and experience of touch. Neuron 42:335–346

Leslie KR, Johnson-Frey SH, Grafton ST 2004 Functional imaging of face and hand imitation: towards a motor theory of empathy. NeuroImage 21:601–607

Lhermitte F, Pillon B, Serdaru MD 1986 Human autonomy and the frontal lobes: I. Imitation and utilization behavior. A neuropsychological study of 75 patients. Ann Neurol 19:326–334

Luria AR 1966 Higher cortical functions in man. Basic Books, New York

Phillips ML, Young AW, Scott SK et al 1998 Neural responses to facial and vocal expressions of fear and disgust. Proc Biol Sci 7:1809–1817

Preston SD, de Waal FBM 2002 Empathy: its ultimate and proximate bases. Behav Brain Sci 25:1–71

Prinz W 2002 Experimental approaches to imitation. In: Meltzoff A, Prinz W (eds) The imitative mind: development, evolution and brain bases. Cambridge University Press, Cambridge, MA

Singer T 2006 The neuronal basis of empathy and fairness. In: Empathy and fairness. Wiley, Chichester (Novartis Found Symp 278), p 20–40

Strayer E 1980 A naturalistic study of empathic behaviors and their relation to affective states and perspective skills in preschool children. Child Dev 51:815–822

Wicker B, Keysers C, Plailly J, Royet JP, Gallese V, Rizzolatti G 2003 Both of us disgusted in My insula: the common neural basis of seeing and feeling disgust. Neuron 40:655–664

DISCUSSION

Van Lange: A nice illustration of empathy is when people are attending movies and empathize with the character to the extent that they start to cry. A specific instance of empathy that struck me was during the first Big Brother reality show in The Netherlands, when one of the participants was looking favourite to leave the house in the next vote. A good friend of mine, who is normal fairly balanced, said he would be willing to pay say 60 Euros if this person could stay in the house: he really empathized with this character. These sorts of emotions are not conscious: there is no analysis of the situation. They just happen. This doesn't involve a lot of cognitive activity.

De Vignemont: I don't claim that we explicitly and consciously analyse the emotional situation. The top–down influences are not available to the subject. You are aware that you empathize, but you are not aware of the reasons why you empathize. Interestingly, in movies you empathize only with one character. We need to understand 'why this one?' and 'why not all of them?'

Blair: You are making direct reference to the more conscious experience of empathy. The problem with that is that we don't have an experimental model of consciousness, so it is not an experimentally tractable question. One of the reasons I never went anywhere near this sort of description is because I knew I'd never be able to have a computational account of it, at least in the short term. It seems to me to be a difficult path to take. You were also shifting from empathy not being automatic, but the neural response or the shared representation being automatic, but we know that this is not correct. The idea used to be that there was an automatic response to, for example, fearful expressions. This has not held up. The degree to which you have that emotional response is determined by the degree to which you attend to the stimulus that generates it. We could flip your argument and say that, yes, we don't empathize all the time, but this is because we are not looking at the face, hands or other triggers. These attentional phenomena can explain this without any complicated alternative processes being invoked.

De Vignemont: I agree that consciousness is a difficult issue to address. Yet empathy involves by definition a conscious emotional reaction similar to the one displayed by the other person. There is a phenomenological aspect that we cannot get rid of. And I think it can be tractable by analysing different situations. For instance, recognition of facial expressions does not elicit a conscious feeling similar to the expression, while seeing someone being hurt does elicit a conscious emotional reaction. By comparing these two situations, we may better understand what is involved in empathy. With regards to your second point, in Tania Singer's experiment, they paid the same amount of attention whether the 'victim' treated the subject fairly or unfairly. Attention cannot explain why she got different results. I don't think we can explain everything by attention, even if it is of course an important factor.

Blair: There are nice models of what attention is about. The Desimone and Duncan model gives a great definition of representational priming leading to attention to particular features of the visual array, driving what the percept is (Desimone & Duncan 1995). Facial expressions are much more powerful than you would anticipate. There is a huge social referencing literature showing that all you need to do is have a novel object in the room, the child is in the room with the mother, looks at the new object, looks at the mother, sees the emotional response of the mother and this determines how the child will respond to the object for ever more. Susan Mineka has very equivalent monkey data (Mineka & Cook 1993).

De Vignemont: I don't say that we are not using facial expressions, just that they don't elicit a strong conscious experience. That is what we are supposed to have in empathy.

Warneken: Your process model started out with the person's observation of the other's emotion and situation, and then went into the shared representation of emotion. Later on you had an arrow going to interpreting or analysing the situation. How much do the first appraisal of the situation and the later analysis differ? Or should this be construed as some kind of feedback loop?

De Vignemont: When you perceive a sensation, you just have for instance the facial expression of pain. This is the first level. At this level, you do not take into account who is in pain or why. This is just the brute observation of pain. It is only at the later stage of the analysis of the emotional event that you process the whole context surrounding this pain. This processing will be influenced by your folk psychology and your folk moral (e.g. children have to be protected), by other beliefs and desires that you have, by your mood and so on. The first level suffices to elicit the shared representation of emotion, but empathy requires taking the context into account.

Warneken: It is not clear to me that the interpretation of the situation comes only later. You could start out with this. Researchers like Doris Bischof-Köhler use this to distinguish between emotional contagion and empathy proper. When the source of information is the facial expression it is more likely that it is personal distress and emotional contagion, versus when it comes through an inference of the situation where it is more likely to be empathy. The self–other differentiation also has to come into the equation, but the first step is already important.

Gergely: There are some potential complications. You have enumerated a set of conditions which, if they are fulfilled, you feel empathy. This may be so. But what would happen if you have a bad day and every five minutes those conditions are satisfied? I don't think you can feel repeatedly, frequently empathic for a long time. Are there further modulating conditions? It is nice that you have pointed out there is no compulsive empathy as a pathological condition. But I have noticed in my family certain older ladies sit in front of the television crying at frequent intervals.

De Vignemont: Perhaps old ladies would be the equivalent of compulsive imitation for empathy! I agree that we cannot repeatedly empathize with different people, but I think we can keep empathizing with the same person over the course of the movie, for example.

C Frith: I have a vague recollection that there are patients who you can manipulate to laugh or cry uncontrollably just by telling them stories.

Moll: Patients with pontine lesions can manifest pathological crying or laughing.

C Frith: But it isn't clear that this is quite the same as empathy.

Gallese: Part of the analysis you made is very helpful, because it helps in pinning down conditions of activation. It is always a challenge to confront our scientific results with philosophers like you. You are helping us in downplaying our enthusiasm, because as soon as we think we have solved a big problem you tell us that it isn't so big. I learned today that the hardest problem is to explain why we don't empathize all the time. I have some doubt that this heavy reliance on the self-conscious notion of what is going on can be used for pinning down what empathy really is. I am trying to find a minimum level of consensus between your idea of empathy and mine. Would you claim that in order to have empathy, a shared representation of the emotion is a necessary but not sufficient condition?

De Vignemont: Yes.

Gallese: So what is missing from this? Is it the selective activation of this mechanism? This mechanism is by default active all the time. To make the activation of this shared representation of emotion the neural equivalent of what empathy is, then what is missing is the condition of activation. I found some problems when you contrasted the voluntary control of imitation with the apparent automaticity of empathy. You said we can't voluntarily control empathy.

De Vignemont: I agree that there is a kind of paradox here. On the one hand we say that imitation is automatic, but we can control it. On the other hand I say that empathy is not automatic, and we cannot control it! This paradox underlines that imitation and empathy follow different principles. Imitation is inhibited most of the time, but sometimes we can voluntarily release it. It is more difficult to control empathy because there is no inhibition that we can just release. To induce empathy, we need the presence of several factors, and we cannot control all of them. Empathy needs to be triggered while imitation just needs to be released. To go back to your first point, I remember in one of your papers you related mirror neurons with empathy (Gallese 2001). I remember you saying that at the phenomenological level we have empathy but at the neural level we have mirror neurons. I think you agree with me that there is something going on at the phenomenological level.

Gallese: My point was that we should keep different levels of description distinct. We shouldn't imbue neurons with intentional properties. They are just fatty bags letting ions come and go. There is no intentional behaviour in a neuron—even a mirror neuron!

Blakemore: In response to your question about whether there are patients who over-empathize, we found a recent case where this occurs. She's not a patient, though; nor is she an old lady. She is a completely normal healthy friend of ours who feels touch when she sees other people being touched. For example, if she sees someone else being touched on their face she feels it on her face as if she is being touched. She has always had this and thought it was completely normal. The way we found her was that I was giving a talk about touch and its perception, and whether this kind of person could exist. She raised her hand and asked whether this wasn't completely normal. We studied her and did an imaging study of how her brain is activated by the observation of touch. We found that her mirror system for touch is overactive. She also feels pain that she observes. She has real problems with horror movies.

C Frith: So that's why she is not a nurse!

De Vignemont: That is very interesting. Empathy is a lot about emotions, and for touch the emotional component is very poor. Pain is more interesting because it is at the borderline between emotion and sensation.

Blakemore: There is a distinction between the automatic empathy for pain which doesn't involve you consciously feeling any emotion or sorrow for the person, and empathy where you cognitively put yourself in the person's shoes. She doesn't report doing this.

Molls: Does she feel the same for good and bad characters?

Blakemore: Yes, it is a bottom–up process.

Singer: The attentional thing doesn't account for everything. In the last experiment I did, the modulation of empathy experiment, subjects were equally attending to the fair and unfair person receiving painful stimulation. The experimental condition was exactly the same. The only difference there was their past history with them and their value judgement about these two players.

Blair: You are talking about the manipulation of whether you liked or disliked the person. The straight attention to the stimulus appeared to be identical, but you got a difference between a strong CS association with a much more rich sensory experience for someone you liked rather than someone you didn't. Therefore you have a more boosted signal that activates a stronger emotional response. I wouldn't have explained your data in attentional terms at all.

Singer: If there would have been much more rich sensory experience for someone you liked this effect should have been controlled by the fact that we are subtracting pain and no pain stimulation for each actor. Thus, your argument does not work here either. Another thing. Why did you say there is no inhibition in empathy? If you could do a time-course analysis with fMRI, you'd want to see whether there is a shared activation of for example pain or touch and then a second re-appraisal process which modulates this activity. It doesn't even have to be top–down inhibition. In my data, I had this dorsolateral prefrontal cortex activity more in men than women when comparing empathic responses to the pain of unfair versus fair players. This activity might reflect modulation of empathic pain responses given men had less of these empathic responses in anterior cingulate cortex (ACC) and AI than women. I don't want to do this claim yet because I would have to design a study specifically to study the Interaction between dorsolateral prefrontal cortex (DLPFC) and anterior insula for example using new methods such as Dynamic causal modelling. But in principle, you could do this kind of experiment to answer the question, and then perhaps you wouldn't have to be as radical as you are. Familiarity, affective link and all these potentially modulatory factors for empathy will have to be explained.

De Vignemont: You are right that there is no temporal dimension in my model. Maybe there is indeed a feedback loop that goes back to the shell representation of emotion and activates it more or less. That could explain some of the results. However, we cannot account for empathy with a purely bottom-up process; we need the top–down input.

Frank: I don't think this was a big part of your case against automatic empathy, but you made a remark about what happens when we see two conflicting emotions in people. Your assessment reminded me of how an economist would look at it: there is a utility function, we have good things and bad things happening, and we just take the net effect, so you are either happy or sad, not both at once. The subjective well-being writers seem to say that this is not the way the happiness and sadness mechanism works. You can experience a happy emotion and a sad emotion at the same time.

C Frith: It seems a pity that consciousness was dismissed. In the imaging work we have no idea whether we are looking at emotional contagion or empathy. We don't know whether it is the conscious or unconscious bit. I don't immediately see how you could separate them out. It would be interesting to study people known as alexithymic, who experience emotions but are not conscious of them in the sense that they don't know what emotion they or having, or even that they are experiencing an emotion at all (Aleman 2005). It would be interesting to know whether these people show empathy. Do they show emotional contagion? The autonomic physiological components of the emotions they experience are larger than normal. There is a suggestion that by being aware of our emotions, things get damped down. This might be part of the mechanism needed for empathizing: you are controlling your own emotions to switch on the one that you think is appropriate to the situation. If real empathy has to be conscious it will be extremely difficult to study it with brain imaging because we should always see the emotional contagion. At the beginning you said that nurses can't be experiencing everything because it would be terrible for them, but by the end it seemed you were saying that they would get all the emotional contagion.

De Vignemont: There would not necessarily be emotional contagion in nurses, but rather an activation of the shared representations of emotion system. Even this activation may be less strong, as noticed by Avenanti et al (2005), who had a nurse among their subjects. She showed a reduced empathetic activity. Perhaps she was habituated to the display of pain.

References

Aleman A 2005 Feelings you can't imagine: towards a cognitive neuroscience of alexithymia. Trends Cogn Sci 9:553–555

Avenanti A, Bueti D, Galati G, Aglioti SM 2005 Transcranial magnetic stimulation highlights the sensorimotor side of empathy for pain. Nat Neurosci 8:955–960

Desimone R, Duncan J 1995 Neural mechanisms of selective visual attention. Annu Rev Neurosci 18:193–222

Gallese V 2001 The 'shared manifold' hypothesis: from mirror neurons to empathy. J Consciousness Stud 8:33–50

Mineka S, Cook M 1993 Mechanisms involved in the observational conditioning of fear. J Exp Psychol Gen 122:23–38

Cooperation through moral commitment

Robert Frank

Cornell University, Ithaca, NY 14853–6201, USA

Abstract. Actions that promote fairness are sometimes consistent with the pursuit of individual self-interest, sometimes not. The diner who leaves a generous tip at a favourite local restaurant, for example, may do so partly out of a sense of obligation to the waiter. But we need not invoke fairness to explain the tip, which is, after all, a prudent investment in obtaining good service in the future. In contrast, narrow self-interest cannot explain why travellers might leave tips in restaurants located along interstate highways. Because it is unlikely that they will ever visit these restaurants again, their failure to tip cannot affect the quality of service they expect to receive in the future. So it is hard to escape the conclusion that concerns about fairness must be implicated when diners tip on the road. Of course, merely to assert the existence of a sense of fairness does not really explain why people often set aside concern for narrow self-interest. It simply raises the more fundamental question of why people have a sense of fairness in the first place. It is this question I will discuss.

2006 Empathy and Fairness. Wiley, Chichester (Novartis Foundation Symposium 278) p 197–215

Imagine having just returned from a crowded concert to discover that you have lost £1000 in cash. The cash had been in an envelope with your name and address on it that apparently fell from your coat pocket while you were at the concert. Do you know anyone not related to you by blood or marriage who you feel certain would return your money? Most people say they do, and for the sake of discussion I will include you in this group. What would make you feel confident that the person you have in mind would return your money?

Note that it is extremely unlikely that you have experienced this situation before. But even if you had, if the friend you named found your money, you would not know that, so there would be no punishment if she kept it. Under the circumstances, returning your money is a strict contradiction of the narrow self-interest model favoured by economists. Most people find it natural to say that the act of returning the money in a situation like this must be motivated by some sort of moral emotion. Thus, you might predict that your friend would return your money because she would feel bad about the prospect of keeping it.

Behaviours that don't fit the self-interest model are actually quite common. Tipping in restaurants can often be rationalized as a self-interested activity, at least in restaurants you visit repeatedly: if you don't tip well, you might not get good service the next time. People resist the temptation to stiff the waiter because the shadow of the future is staring at them. But if it is a restaurant that you don't expect to visit again, this explanation doesn't work. Yet people tip at about the same rate at such restaurants (Bodvarsson & Gibson 1994).

An editor once sent me a paper for review that purported to confirm economic theory's prediction about tipping rates in different types of restaurants. Most of the restaurants in the authors' sample were ones frequented primarily by local diners, but one served a predominantly out-of-town clientele. And sure enough, the tipping rate was lower in that one restaurant. But the difference was extremely small—something like 13.5 percent as opposed to a little more than 15 percent in the other restaurants. I wrote back that this was indeed an interesting result but for the opposite reason, since the self-interest model predicts a tipping rate near zero for the restaurant patronized mostly by non-locals.

Some explain the apparent anomaly of tipping on the road as a simple consequence of information costs. When people eat out, it is mostly at local restaurants, and they know from experience that tipping is in their interest in such restaurants. They may not take the trouble to calculate that optimal tipping behaviour might be different for out-of-town restaurants. This explanation suggests that when someone is told that he could get away without leaving a tip when dining on the road, he should seem grateful for the information and modify his behaviour accordingly. But this reaction is uncommon. Most people find it odd that economic models might predict no tipping on the road. When pressed, they will say something to the effect that if the waiter did a good job, they would feel bad about not having left a tip.

Again, tipping on the road is not an isolated anomaly. For example, when sociologists drop wallets containing small amounts of cash on sidewalks in New York, about half come back with the cash intact (Hornstein 1976). There was not enough cash in the wallets for anyone to have expected a reward commensurate with the time it takes to wait in line at the post office to send it back.

The Falklands War is another good example. The British could have bought the Falklanders out—giving each family, say, a castle in Scotland and a generous pension for life—for far less than the cost of sending their forces to confront the Argentineans. Instead they incurred a great cost in treasure and lives. Yet few in the UK opposed the decision to fight for the desolate South Atlantic islands. It wasn't that there was a far-flung empire that Britain needed to signal its willingness to defend. You could say that Margaret Thatcher gained politically by responding as she did, but this begs the question of why voters preferred retaliation to inaction. When pressed, most people speak in terms of the nation's honour being at stake.

People rescue others in distress even at great peril to themselves; they donate bone marrow to strangers. Such behaviours are in tension with the standard rational choice model favoured by economists. They seem to be motivated by moral sentiments. Where do these sentiments come from? One version of the economist's rational choice model, called the present-aim model, holds people are rational if they are efficient in their pursuit of whatever goals they happen to hold when they act. Thus, people are said to leave tips when dining on the road because they get a warm glow from doing so. This sounds descriptive, but why do people get a warm glow from tipping as opposed to not tipping?

Adam Smith said that moral sentiments were endowed in us by the creator for the good of society. It is true that society works better if people have these moral sentiments. But as Darwin emphasized, selection occurs not at the society level but at the level of the individual organism. Moral sentiments motivate people to occur costs that they could avoid in many cases, so on what basis might these sentiments have been favoured by natural selection? The mechanism I am going to explore is from Tom Schelling's work on the difficulties people face when confronted with what are called commitment problems (Schelling 1960).

The example he used was the kidnapper who seizes a victim and then gets cold feet. He wants to set the victim free but knows that, once freed, the victim will reveal the kidnapper's identity to the police. So the kidnapper reluctantly decides he must kill the victim. The victim doesn't want to die and wants to promise not to go to the police. The problem is that both know that once he is out the door, his motive for keeping that promise will vanish. Schelling suggests a solution. If there is some evidence of a crime that the victim has committed, he can share that evidence with the kidnapper, which will create a bond ensuring his silence. The evidence of the victim's crime is a commitment device that makes an otherwise empty promise credible.

Schelling's basic insight can be applied to show why a trustworthy person might be able to prosper even in highly competitive market settings. Suppose you have a business that is doing so well that you know it would thrive in a similar town 300 miles distant. The problem is that because you can't monitor the manager who would run this business, he would be free to cheat you. Suppose a managerial candidate promises to manage honestly. You must then decide whether to open the branch office. If you do and your employee manages honestly, you each come out very well—say, £1000 each better than the status quo. But if the manager cheats, you will lose £500 on the deal and he will gain £1500. The relevant payoffs for each of the options are thus as summarized in Figure 1.

If you open the outlet, the manager finds himself on the top branch of the decision tree, where he faces a choice between cheating and not. If he cheats his payoff is £1500; if not, his payoff is only £1000. Standard rational choice models assume that managers in these situations will be self-interested in the narrow sense. If that

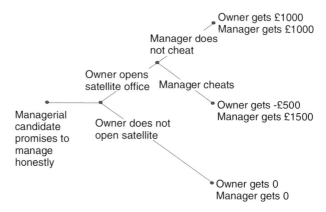

Owner gets £1000
Manager gets £1000
Manager does
not cheat

Owner opens
satellite office   Manager cheats

Managerial
candidate   Owner gets -£500
promises to   Owner does not   Manager gets £1500
manage   open satellite
honestly

Owner gets 0
Manager gets 0

FIG. 1.   The branch-outlet problem.

is your belief, you predict that the manager will cheat, which means your payoff will be =£500. And since that is worse than the payoff of zero you would get if you didn't open the branch outlet, your best bet is not to open it. The pity is that this means a loss to both you and the manager relative to what could have been achieved had you opened the branch outlet and the manager ran it honestly.

Now suppose you can identify a managerial candidate who would be willing to pay £10 000 to avoid the guilt he would feel if he cheated you. Needless to say, using a financial penalty as a proxy for guilt feelings would be inappropriate in normative discourse. We would not say, for example, that it's OK to cheat as long as you gain enough to compensate for the resulting feelings of guilt. But the formulation does nonetheless capture an important element of behaviour. People respond to incentives, and are less likely to cheat when the penalties are higher.

In any event, it is clear how this simple change transforms the equilibrium of the game. If the manager cheats, his payoff is not £1500 but =£8500 (after the £10 000 psychological burden is deducted). So, if you open the branch outlet, the manager will choose to manage honestly, and both he and you come out ahead. If you could identify a trustworthy person in this situation, he or she would not be at a disadvantage. On the contrary, both you and the manager would clearly profit.

Note, however, that the managerial candidate won't be hired unless his taste for honesty is observable. Thus an honest candidate who is not believed to be honest fares worse than a dishonest candidate who is believed to be honest. The first doesn't even get hired. The second not only gets the job but also the fruits of cheating the owner.

Imagine a mutation that caused trustworthy people to be born with an identifying mark, such as a 'c' on the forehead (for 'cooperator'). Then the problem would

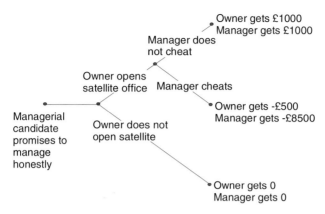

FIG. 2.   The branch-outlet problem with an honest manager.

be solved. In such a world, the trustworthy types would drive the untrustworthy types to extinction. If the two types are costlessly distinguishable, the only equilibrium is one with pure trustworthy types in the population (Frank 1988, chapter 3).

In general, though, it is costly to figure out who is who. So people would not be vigilant in their choice of trading partners in an environment in which everyone was trustworthy. It wouldn't pay, just as it wouldn't pay to buy an expensive security system for your apartment if you lived in a neighbourhood in which there had never been a burglary. Thus, a population consisting exclusively of trustworthy types could not be an evolutionarily stable equilibrium. Given reduced levels of vigilance, untrustworthy types could invade such a population. So if character traits are costly to observe, the only sustainable equilibrium is one where there is a mixed population consisting of both honest and dishonest individuals.

How might a signal of trustworthiness have emerged in the first place? Even if the first trustworthy person bore some observable marker, no one else would have had any idea what it would have meant. Nico Tinbergen argued that if there is ever a signal of any trait, its emergence in the first instance must be a complete accident (Tinbergen 1952). That is, if a trait is accompanied by an observable marker, the link between the trait and the marker had to have arisen by chance. For example, the dung beetle escapes predators by resembling the dung on which it feeds. How did it get to look like this? Unless it just happened to look enough like a fragment of dung to have fooled the most near-sighted predator out there, the first step toward a more dung-like appearance couldn't have been favoured by natural selection. As Stephen Jay Gould asked, 'Can there be any advantage in looking 5% like a turd?' (Gould 1977, p 104) The problem is that no one would be fooled. So how does the threshold level of resemblance reached? It has to be by some accidental link between appearance and surroundings. But once such a link exists, then selection can begin to shape appearance systematically.

Similarly, we may ask, 'How could a moral sentiment could have emerged if no one initially knew the significance of its accompanying marker?' One hypothesis is suggested by the logic of the iterated prisoner's dilemma (Frank 1988, chapter 4). There is no difficulty explaining why a self-interested person would cooperate in an iterated prisoner's dilemma. You get a string of cooperations going if you are a tit-for-tat player and happen to pair with another such player on the first round (Rapoport & Chammah 1965). For this reason, even Attila the Hun, lacking any moral sentiments, would want to cooperate on the first move of an iterated prisoner's dilemma. The problem is that if you cooperate on the first move, you are forgoing some gain in the present moment, although you expect to more than recoup that sacrifice in the future. Still, there is a time discount factor that must be engaged. What we know is that organisms in general aren't very good at this: they tend to favour small immediate rewards over even much larger long-term rewards (Ainslie 1992).

If you were endowed with a moral sentiment that made you feel bad when you cheated your partner, even if no one could see that you had that sentiment, this would make you better able to resist the temptation to cheat in the first round. And that, in turn, would enable you generate a reputation for being a cooperative person, which would be clearly to your advantage.

Moral emotions may thus have two separate roles. They are impulse control devices. The activation of these emotions, like other forms of brain activation, may be accompanied by involuntary external symptoms that are observable. If so, the observable symptoms over time could have become associated in others' minds with the presence of the moral sentiments. And once that association was recognized, the moral emotions would be able to play a second role—namely, that of helping people solve one-shot prisoner's dilemmas. The symptoms themselves can then be further refined by natural selection because of their capacity to help others identify people who might be good partners in one-shot dilemmas.

How do you communicate something to another individual who has reason to be sceptical of what you are saying? Suppose, for example, that a toad meets a rival and both want the same mate. Among animals generally, the smaller of two rivals defers to the larger, thereby avoiding a costly fight that he would be likely to lose anyway. Rival toads, however, often encounter one another at night, making visual assessment difficult. What they do is croak at one another, and the toad with the higher-pitched croak defers. The idea is that the lower your croak the bigger you are on average. So it's prudent to defer to the lower croaker. This example illustrates the costly-to-fake principle: 'I'll believe you not because you *say* you are a big toad, but rather because you are using a signal that is difficult to present unless you really *are* a big toad' (Frank 1988, chapter 6).

It's the same when dogs face off: they seem to follow an algorithm of deferring to the larger dog. Consider the drawings in Fig. 3, taken from Charles Darwin's 1872 book, *The Expression of Emotion in Man and Animals*. The left panel portrays a dog that is confronting a rival. Darwin argued that we reliably infer what is going on emotionally in this dog's brain by observing the numerous elements of its posture are so serviceable in the combat mode: the dog's hackles are raised, its fangs are bared, its ears are pricked, its eyes wide open and alert, its body poised to spring forward. Darwin reasoned that any dog that had to go through a conscious checklist to manifest these postural elements one by one would be too slow on the draw to compete effectively against a rival in whom the entire process was activated autonomously by the relevant emotional arousal. That link, he concluded, provides a window into the dog's brain.

Darwin argued that there are similar systems in humans (Darwin 1872). Certain expressions, for example, spring unbidden to the human face in the presence of triggering emotions, yet are extremely difficult to present when those emotions are absent. People raised in different cultural traditions around the world can readily identify the schematic expression portrayed in Fig. 4 as one corresponding to emotions such as sadness or concern. As Paul Ekman and his colleagues have shown, most people are unable to reproduce this expression on command (Ekman 1985). Various emotions have their characteristic signatures.

In the argument I am attempting to advance, sympathy or empathy is an especially important moral emotion. How do you know whether someone will treat your interests with respect when he has an opportunity to cheat you with no possibility of being punished? You would probably feel more secure in this situation if you felt you were dealing with someone with whom you enjoyed a strong sympathetic bond. Recall the thought experiment asking whether you felt you could name someone you felt sure would return a lost envelope full of cash.

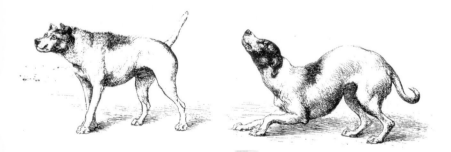

FIG. 3.   Observable correlates of emotional states.

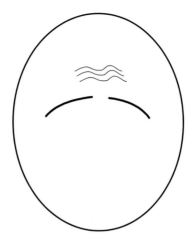

FIG. 4.   The characteristic expression of sadness or concern.

I have been talking thus far as if there were good people and bad people, with some mixture of these two pure types comprising the entire population. In fact, it is far more complicated: we have all done something decent and we have all cheated at one point or another. The question is, under what conditions do we cheat? Evidence suggests that we are far less likely to cheat others with whom we enjoy strong sympathetic bonds.

Such bonds appear to form as a result of a complex dance that plays out among people over time. Many aspects of this dance are mechanical. Certain actions affect us even though there is no obvious reason they should. For example, I set my watch 10 minutes ahead because it gets me to appointments on time more often. This trick works even though I can always tell the correct time by just subtracting 10 minutes from the time indicated by my watch. Yet the image on my watch gets into my brain through multiple pathways. Along one pathway, it goes to a part of my brain that makes the 10-minute adjustment. But along another pathway, it goes somewhere in the limbic system, where the uncorrected image makes me feel anxious about my risk of being late. The formation of sympathetic bonds among people entails many processes that are much like this one (for a richly insightful discussion of the process by which sympathetic bonds form, see Sally 2000).

If we show you Chinese ideographs while you are pulling on a lever, and we show you different ideographs while you are pushing on a lever—and this is subliminal so you don't even know you are seeing the images—then later when we show you the two sets of ideographs, you like the ones that you saw when you were pulling but not those when you were pushing the lever (Cacciopo et al 1993).

Is a cartoon funny? It is difficult to predict what will provoke someone to laughter. But if you see the cartoon when you have a pencil in your teeth you will rate it as funnier than if you don't have a pencil in your teeth. Having a pencil in your mouth causes the muscles of the face to move in ways similar to the ones that produce a smile (Strack et al 1988).

There is also what psychologists call the mere exposure effect: we show you Chinese characters subliminally, some of them frequently, others infrequently. Then we show you a list of all the characters you were shown and ask which ones you prefer. Invariably, people voice a preference for the characters they were shown most frequently.

Preference for the familiar extends to persons. We sometimes prefer the company of a person we know even if we have good reason to believe that we ought to prefer another person we don't know as well.

Every stimulus we confront generates a positive or negative initial valence. This is true of words, objects, persons, every stimulus. The more another person is like you, the more likely you are to experience a positive valence upon meeting that person. Reputation matters for obvious reasons. Physical attractiveness matters distressingly much: if you are interacting with an attractive person you are much more likely to experience a positive valence than if it is a person you find unattractive (Eagly et al 1991). Expressiveness is another thing that generates positive valence. The initial exchange matters a lot: if you had a good first exchange this sets a tone that tends to persist.

Once the initial valence for a person is established, a subliminal cognitive filter screens subsequent information about that person in a biased way. It tries to confirm your initial impression. So when you receive ambiguous signals after your first encounter you interpret them positively if your initial impression was positive, and negatively if your initial impression was negative. It is not that first impressions are immune from revision. Although you tend to ignore data that are contradictory, if they are salient enough, you take them into account.

Also implicated in the process is sympathetic mimicry, a rich application of the motor neuron system (Bavelas et al 1986). When you are interacting with someone, you tend to mimic automatically what that person does. Chartrand and Bargh have taught some of their research assistants to suppress the tendency to mimic others (Chartrand & Bargh 1999). The assistants will then have conversations with undergraduate subjects. With a control group, they don't suppress the mimicry tendency, but with the treatment group they do. In exit interviews, treatment subjects typically say they didn't like their conversation partners. Control subjects voice the opposite opinion.

If you live with someone for a long time, you end up mimicking that person's expressions repeatedly, which may help explain why husbands and wives come to resemble one another over time. In one experiment, investigators cut wedding photos in half and asked subjects to guess which men were married to which women. Their guesses did not surpass chance accuracy. But when they cut 25th-anniversary photographs in half, subjects were able to match spouses with significantly better than chance accuracy (Zajonc et al 1987).

Intensity of interaction is another predictor of the strength of sympathetic bonds. Army units that are heavily bombarded in combat stay in touch with each other for many more years than units that aren't (Elder & Clipp 1988). Heavy-weight boxers John Tunney and Jack Dempsey had three brutal championship bouts in the early years of the 20th century. They were said not to like one another. Yet they stayed in touch over the years. They seemed to have a bond that emerged from that process (Heimer 1969).

This is necessarily a rough sketch of the process by which sympathetic bonds form. It is a process laden with contingency. When you have a commitment problem to solve, you pick somebody who you think cares about you. People are critical of George Bush for giving jobs to cronies. But all leaders do that, and for good reason. Bush's particular problem has been that many of his cronies were incompetent. The idea that you would pick someone well known to you is intelligible; it is a sensible thing to do. In the end, the question is whether we can identify who will cheat and who won't.

Tom Gilvich, Dennis Regan and I have done some experiments on this (Frank et al 1993b). We examined the choice of people who played prisoner's dilemma games after brief interactions with two partners. Subjects talked with one another for 30 minutes before going into separate rooms to fill out forms on which they indicated, for each partner, whether they were going to cooperate or defect. They also recorded their predictions of what each partner would do when playing with them. Each subject's payoff was then the sum of the payoffs from the relevant cells of the two games, plus a random term, so no one knew after the fact who had done what.

Almost 74% of the people cooperated in this pure one-shot prisoner's dilemma. This finding is completely unpredicted by the standard self-interest model. But other empirical studies have also found high cooperation rates in dilemmas when subjects were allowed to communicate. Our particular concern was with whether subjects could predict how each of their specific partners would play. When someone predicted that a partner would cooperate there was an 81% likelihood of cooperation (as opposed to the 74% base rate). On the defection side, the base rate was just over 26%, but partners who were predicted to defect had a defection rate of almost 57%. This seems an astonishingly good prediction on the basis of just 30 minutes of informal conversation.

Ernst Fehr and Urs Fischbacher have also done some experiments in which he found that people are better than chance at predicting who will cheat (Fehr & Fischbacher 2005). Fehr and Fischbacher noted that if subjects chose partners on the basis of their predictions, cooperators would have earned a smaller payoff, on average, than defectors. From this they concluded that our predictions of cooperation are not sufficiently accurate to have supported the evolution of trustworthiness. But this conclusion does not follow (Frank 2005). If trustworthiness is to be favoured by natural selection, some people must be able to identify its presence in others. It is not necessary that everyone, on the basis of limited exposure, be able to identify whether randomly selected strangers are trustworthy. Thus, in choosing a manager for a branch outlet, you would normally pick someone with whom you have sufficient time to permit a much firmer character assessment. Even if only a limited number of others can identify you as trustworthy, you become an attractive candidate for interactions that require trust.

Let's go back to the original thought experiment with the envelope of £1000. How did you pick the person who you thought would return your money if she found it? Typically it is someone with whom the sympathy dance has unfolded over an extended period. The feeling is that you know enough about this person to say that if she found your money, she wouldn't feel right about keeping it.

Throughout their careers, many economists employ self-interest models to predict how people will behave. Does this affect their own behaviour? The answer seems to be yes. In the same experiments in which we investigated whether people could predict who would cooperate, Gilovich, Regan, and I found that economics majors were far more likely to defect (Frank et al 1993a). This difference could be either a selection effect, a training effect, or some mix of the two. We found evidence that economics training itself has some effect. There is a general humanizing trend that seems to be at work in the university as students progress through school. The underclassmen defect at a much higher rate than juniors and seniors. This humanizing trend was not observed among the economics majors.

To say that trustworthiness could be an evolutionarily stable strategy is not to say that everyone is primed to cooperate all the time. Opportunism of the sort predicted by self-interest models is abundant. Yet the prospects for sustaining cooperation in one-shot dilemmas are not as bleak as many economists seem to think. Many people are willing to set aside self interest to promote the common good. Even if moral emotions are unobservable by others, they can still help you to be patient in repeated prisoner's dilemmas. But if others recognize you to be a decent person, there are all sorts of ways in which you are valuable. If you are in business, your boss is likely to have a firm opinion about whether you'd be the sort of person to return the lost £1000 if you found it. You'd like him to think that you'd return it. Perhaps the best way to get him to think that is actually to be the kind of person who would return it.

References

Ainslie G 1992 Picoeconomics. Cambridge University Press, New York

Bavelas JB, Black A, Lemery CR, Mullett J 1986 I show how you feel: Motor mimicry as a communicative Act. J Pers Soc Psychol 50:322–329

Bodvarsson OB, Gibson WA 1994 Gratuities and customer appraisal of service: evidence from Minnesota restaurants. Journal of Socioeconomics 23:287–302

Cacioppo JT, Priester JR, Berntson GG 1993 Rudimentary determinants of attitudes, II: Arm flexion and extension have differential effects on attitudes. J Pers Soc Psychol 65:5–17

Chartrand TL, Bargh JA 1999 The unbearable automaticity of being. Am Psychol 54:462–479

Darwin C 1965; 1872 The expression of emotions in man and animals. University of Chicago Press, Chicago

Elder GH, Clipp EC 1988 Wartime losses and social bonding: Influence across 40 years in men's lives. Psychiatry 51:177–198

Eagly AH, Ashmore RD, Makhijani MG, Longo LC 1991 What is beautiful is good, but. . .: A meta-analytic review of research on the physical attractiveness stereotype. Psychol Bull 110:109–128

Ekman P 1985 Telling Lies. W. W. Norton, New York

Fehr E, Fischbacher U 2005 Altruists with Green Beards. Analyse & Kritik 27:73–84

Frank RH 1988 Passions within reason. W. W. Norton, New York

Frank RH, Gilovich T, Regan D 1993a Does studying economics inhibit cooperation? J Econ Perspect 7 Spring 159–171

Frank RH, Gilovich T, Regan DT 1993b The evolution of one-shot cooperation. Ethol Sociobiol 14:247–256

Frank RH 2005 Altruists with green beards: Still kicking? Analyse & Kritik 1·85–96

Gould SJ 1977 Ever since Darwin. W. W. Norton, New York

Heimer M 1969 The Long Count. Athenum, New York

Hornstein H 1976 Cruelty and kindness, Englewood Cliffs, Prentice Hall, NJ

Rapoport A, Chammah A 1965 Prisoner's Dilemma. University of Michigan Press, Ann Arbor

Sally D 2000 A general theory of sympathy, mind-reading, and social interaction, with an application to the prisoners' dilemma. Social Science Information 39:567–634

Schelling TC 1960 The strategy of conflict. Oxford University Press, New York

Smith A 1966; 1759 The theory of moral sentiments. Kelley, New York

Strack F, Martin LL, Stepper S 1988 Inhibiting and facilitating conditions of the human smile: a nonobtrusive test of the facial feedback hypothesis. J Pers Soc Psychol 54:768–776

Tinbergen N 1952 Derived activities: their causation, biological significance, and emancipation during evolution. Q Rev Biol 27:1–32

Zajonc RB, Adelmann PK, Murphy ST, Niedenthal PM 1987 Convergence in the physical appearance of spouses. Motivation and Emotion 11:335–346

DISCUSSION

Van Lange: I liked the latter study very much. People are willing to pay a lot for hiding information. Sometimes people want to do this for self-protective reasons. This has a nice link with the literature on noise in social dilemmas. Sometimes people seek out uncertainty for those reasons. With regard to mimicry, there is recent evidence that if you are a waiter and you mimic the customer you get greater tips.

Frank: This prompts the question: do we really want people to know all this?

Moll: There is an interesting recent paper on anonymous public games with a number of interventions (Messer et al 2005). One is that people chat ('cheap talk'), and this increased the contributions to the public good, but contributions are not stable over time. In another treatment, participants chat and vote, thereby making commitments before playing the game. Although the game is totally anonymous (i.e. there is no way to know who is actually sticking to the agreement or not), in this situation there is stable cooperation over time. Perhaps newly developed norms that are agreed upon provide a strong incentive for people. It would be very interesting to understand why and how people stick to these norms.

Frank: So they state their intentions? That helps in all one-shot prisoner's dilemma games I've done. While in game theory this would just be cheap talk, in fact it seems to matter. To say you are going to cooperate and then defect would be an extra hurdle for most people.

Moll: It seems that the voting procedure, in addition to cheap talk, boost even more cooperative behaviour, adding stability over time. Could this be compared to a new cultural norm?

Frank: The whole issue of how these norms become established is attracting a lot of study now, but we still don't know much about them.

Silk: This account resonates with my intuition about how people behave. But why does this mechanism only operate in humans? Chimpanzees cooperate and they do better if they cooperate, and there are lots of contexts in which you could imagine that other animals would profit from this ability. How come they don't have it?

Frank: Frans de Waal claims that he sees precursors of this in chimps. If you see how fragile it is in humans, it is not surprising to think that the emergence of this behaviour requires a whole lot of things to happen.

Silk: It is a fragile process, but we have succeeded in sustaining cooperation despite this.

Frank: The moment the system relaxes things change. There is a tendency for it to unravel very quickly unless there are controls in place in the background.

Silk: But people return wallets.

Call: A key question is what qualifies as a precursor. What would we take as evidence of something perhaps homologous to what is seen in humans?

Frank: Distress at the pain of another is observed in chimps, isn't it?

Brosnan: It depends on who you talk to. There are certainly anecdotes of instances that look like reactions to pain. There is an example involving a gorilla at the San Diego zoo. A new female gorilla got a shock reaching her hand through some electrified wire to get some grass on the other side. The next day she saw an older female gorilla who knew how to reach through the fence without getting shocked doing the same, and the younger female cringed as if she was anticipating the other's pain even though the older female received no shock. There are lots of anecdotal examples but there haven't been any studies demonstrating consistent responses to the distress of others, partially because it is unethical to create distress to see what happens.

Silk: When people have looked and tried to elicit that kind of responding they haven't been successful. There have been experiments which have shown that mothers do not prevent their infants from eating things that made them sick themselves. If the mother knows that there is a scary thing in a box, does she intervene when an infant approaches it? No.

Frank: You wouldn't need moral sentiments to get that to happen. There would be such a close kin bond that if they could cognitively manage it, they would want to intervene whether they felt like doing it or not.

Montague: It doesn't have to be consistent to be a prototype. All the traits that we have now weren't systematically represented in populations that preceded us.

Brosnan: It seems to me that most of the examples of what has proposed to be empathy occur in high emotional intensity situations. It may be that among the chimpanzees, many situations don't have high enough emotional arousal for empathic responses. The other question is whether it is empathy in the same way that humans experience it.

Call: Is it empathy or emotional contagion?

Silk: One builds on the other. The question is where we get the ratchet effect phylogenetically.

Brosnan: Chimps certainly cooperate, both in the field and in the lab, but not at the same level of complexity as is seen in humans. Perhaps they don't have a need for a system that allows such complex cooperation to evolve. It seems to us that it would make sense, but perhaps the gains are so little that it is not worth the cost.

Frank: There is a parallel account for the emergence of anger. If someone commits aggression against you and it is an ongoing relationship, then it is prudent for you to retaliate, even if the cost of retaliating now is bigger than what you lost in the first place, just because the value of signalling that you are not to be messed with will repay that loss over the course of time. This is still an impulse-control problem, because you have to endure the big cost up front in order to get that string of benefits. If you are angry and want to retaliate, this helps you get over the impulse-control hurdle. I don't know whether in animals the fury reaction in response to aggression is observed.

Silk: I think dominance is like that. It is normally not about anything. It is about setting things up so that later no one wants to usurp you.

Brosnan: Like chimpanzees in the field learning to use empty kerosene cans to get dominance. But I'm not sure that the shadow of the future looms as large in chimpanzees as it does in humans. I am not sure they can plan ahead to the extent that we can, which could affect the moral compassion argument.

Blair: I had the same worry about the precursor. With regard to the response, when you were talking about empathy in the chimps you were talking about the personal distress issue and a planned response to another animal's distress. This is a lot more complicated than whether they were bothered by another animal's distress. I am assuming that chimpanzees make a noise when they are in pain. This will have a communicatory purpose. Rats make a noise when they are in pain and it is such a spectacular cue that it has been used as an inducer for a rat model of post-traumatic stress disorder (PTSD). Again, the rats don't go round trying to cuddle each other afterwards, but with regards to the basic response to another animal in pain, I think this is too primitive a precursor to relate it to the things you were talking about.

Frank: Josep Call, what cues would you rely on if you had to predict whether someone would return your lost money?

Call: Believe it or not, one of the cues would be does the person need the money?

Frank: If no, then he will return it?

Call: Yes, but it is not just this. Cues would be on other occasions when this person had the opportunity to defect, did they?

Frank: If on past occasions you knew whether he defected, then it is not really a one-shot game.

Montague: What other data would you use to establish a reliability metric about the likelihood of him returning the money?

Frank: The argument is that if you were just a nasty guy and were in a repeated prisoner's dilemma, then you would cooperate. So why would seeing someone do that be diagnostic of what would happen with the found wallet?

Montague: I don't understand. Why wouldn't you use even a one-shot interaction in the past as a datum? Your repeated history with a person is nothing but a repeated game of a heterogeneous sort.

Frank: But if two nasty people cooperated in repeated games, what do I learn unless there is something like this process whereby we become bonded to one another.

Montague: First movers in one-shot games will routinely give money. Mechanistically, when this is probed experimentally people have this risk mitigated. A rational actor would never start a one-shot game with you, yet when you test this, most people do. A mechanism has been built into your head to mitigate the risk that would otherwise sit there in a game theoretic sense.

Silk: Cooperating is not a rational model. If everyone behaved the way economists did, it would be rational enough to cooperate.

Montague: No, it is rational to cooperate if there is a likelihood of multiple interactions or rounds.

Silk: No, even in a one-shot. If people behave the way people behave in one-shot games then it is rational to cooperate.

Frank: No, because defecting is a dominant strategy. If you cooperate I do better if I defect.

Silk: But not if people don't defect.

Van Lange: Repeated interactions are a trust building process from a psychological perspective.

Montague: If there is risk on each decision. If I give you $20 and the options you have for paying me back are only that you can give me $15, I learn nothing. If you may keep it all and give me nothing such that there is a risk that I lose, then I get data from that.

Frank: If I have to take an active step to return the money, then that does influence people's perceptions, even though it shouldn't.

Montague: There's a risk of a loss there, so I get data. If you either always give me a loss or always give a gain, I learn nothing.

Frank: It could be a situation where if I were a self-interested rational person you would perceive no risk of me not paying you back. It would be in my interest to pay you back and so you would predict that I would. Perhaps you learn just that I am a self-interested rational person.

Montague: That isn't the way humans behave.

Frank: That's what I'm saying, but how do we account for the staying power of people who don't behave that way?

Montague: We are learning machines. We have to probe the world at risk in order to get information back from the world. I will be willing to take a chance to gain information that will be valuable to me in the future. It plugs straight into a learning mechanism.

Call: Would you choose a stranger with whom you have not interacted to trust to return the money to you? Or would you choose someone with whom you have interacted repeatedly?

Frank: The latter, of course.

Brosnan: If it were a stranger with whom you have never interacted before, there would be aspects to their behaviour, or knowledge of what they did, that might make them more trustworthy.

Call: That is getting data.

Montague: It's an inference problem, then. They are proxies for what they are likely to be like.

Gergely: I want to raise the question of differential types of cues that go into this familiarization. There are some that are directly useful and give data precisely for the domain to which you want to apply it. Then there are cues like the chameleon effect. There is no perceptual link here. These types of spontaneous cues that do build trust and cooperation may serve more directly another function. Establishing common ground and familiarity are within group-types of cues you can count on to decrease the likelihood of aggression against you. The more common ground you have the less likely is aggression.

Van Lange: It could be more prosocial than non-aggressive.

Gergely: It is a different function and it may flow over into decisions about trust. Last year we were at a conference at a beautiful coastline in North Carolina. One of the researchers was speaking about sharing and common ground. He reported that in the morning he went out and saw dolphins jumping out of the water. There was a total stranger there also and he felt the inclination to share the experience with him. This was supposed to be a spontaneously driven instinctive sharing with a total stranger. There is another possibility that there is a spontaneous drive in humans to build up as fast as possible a common ground with others. My intuition is that the primary function of this is more of a defence against the possibility of being physically aggressed.

Frank: That seems analogous with what I said. If you want me to incur costs on your behalf hoping some day you will do the same, then you have to want me to trust you.

Van Lange: Interestingly, it takes very little to get some trust. There is one classic study that if you are on the beach and you ask someone to keep an eye on your radio, this person is then less likely to steal it than if you don't ask them.

Montague: It is fragile. There is a price point. If you turn the number up then all the rules start morphing at some point.

Silk: In your thought experiment, if you asked if you knew anyone who would send the wallet back to a complete stranger, this seems to me a different question. It highlights that some of this is about the disposition or nature of individuals: what is interesting is that we don't think about people only in the context of their interactions with us. We think that their interactions with us are predictive of their relationships with others. This is an interesting feature. Why don't we behave differently to some people than to others?

Frank: You could ask the separate question: Do you know someone who would return a stranger's wallet? People can usually identify people in that category, too. I chose returning your own wallet because this question is so much easier.

Montague: In hunter–gatherers what is the relative fraction of one-shot versus repeated interactions? It seems to me one-shot is a minority behaviour to be probing these algorithms.

Frank: The fact that an interaction is with someone you know doesn't mean that it is one-shot.

Montague: What I mean is did the mechanisms evolve in the context of having to keep a history?

Frank: So the question is, is there an opportunity for you to cheat someone with a sufficiently low probability of detection that it is in effect a one-shot interaction?

If you come across a food source, for example, can you conceal it and no one will know?

Silk: In evolutionary psychology, the conventional answer is that it is all repeated interactions with familiar individuals. But I don't think this is ethnographically correct.

Montague: Are populations large enough that one-shot interactions are common but still a minority occurrence?

Silk: Certainly, they are not as common as in our societies. I call this the 'people are more stupid than vervet monkeys' hypothesis. Many kinds of primates carefully differentiate between kin, reciprocating partners and everyone else, and they live in groups of 30. This idea that we are not smart enough to figure out the difference between a one-shot interaction and a repeated interaction is not plausible.

Montague: What you said speaks poignantly to these one-shot ultimatum games that people have been playing. What you are probing is ambiguous because you don't have a good estimate of the prior in that person's head. Is this person thinking it is a one-shot? There are all these proxies in those settings. These ultimatum games are a one-shot. They are confusing to me because I don't know where they start: what is the person doing when I interact with them? Does the cover story set them up one way and not another?

Frank: One thing is that evolutionary psychologists say is that we are so used to doing multi-period games that we are wired to think in these terms. It is not worth calculating whether it is a one-shot game or not because the odds of it being one are low enough that we don't go there.

Montague: So you think that these ultimatum games are being perceived by the people doing them as multiple games?

Frank: Yes, by some people. In the tipping on the road case, you could say that people tip on the road because they are in the habit of behaving this way in restaurants. If you tell them that no harm will come to them by not tipping, you can do the computation for them and they then don't seem to change their behaviour.

Brosnan: If you think of one-shot interactions as being situations where you can get away with something, even chimpanzees change their food calling depending on how much food they find and whether or not there is an audience. If they find a small amount of food that they can eat quickly, they will eat it without making any food calls (Brosnan & de Waal 2003). There are a number of explanations for this. They can distinguish between a situation where they have the opportunity to interact.

Montague: I am not saying that humans can't distinguish, rather that there is now a large body of experimental evidence in behavioural economics on one-shot games, where step 1 has not been disambiguated with regard to this issue I'm bringing up. It makes it very hard to understand what the outcome will be.

Silk: This is a real dispute. Many people make the point you are raising.

Montague: It would be easy to fix. You could pin the game down more, and assure yourself of the priors of the participants for this game.

Frank: In the prisoner's dilemma experiments we did, we asked people what the consequence would be of different combinations of choices. They got the right answer. They knew the right payoff, for example, when asked what happens if they defect and the other cooperates.

Van Lange: If you ask people what they prefer, they don't always prefer the rational option. Most people prefer the cell where both cooperate in a single-trial prisoner's dilemma. Perhaps this is because it is a fair solution. This is something that they place value on. Sometimes they also anticipate regret that if they defect, it is not pleasant for the other person.

Montague: There is also the issue of reputation in the eyes of the experimenter.

Silk: Many of these experiments are double blind. It's hard to do.

References

Brosnan SF, de Waal FBM 2003 Regulation of vocalizations by chimpanzees finding food in the presence or absence of an audience. Evol Communicat 4:211–224

Messer KD, Kaiser HM, Schulze WD 2005 Context and voluntary contributions: an experimental analysis of communication, voting, and status quo bias. *http://www.business.appstate.edu/departments/economics/workshoppapers/Schulze.pdf*

FINAL DISCUSSION

U Frith: I want to bring up the idea of priors. Earlier on we discussed the idea of whether there could be an identifiable sign of whether or not you are a trustworthy person. This would make a huge difference. There are perhaps mechanisms in place that amount to prejudice or stereotyping: as soon as you see a person, you have an immediate idea about their trustworthiness on a non-objective basis.

C Frith: It's whether or not you wear a tie!

Frank: There are costly-to-fake signals. Someone mentioned the choice of job. How do you know how much a person cares about the moral high ground? You can look at the pay differential across jobs that are in virtually every respect identical, except for what could be described as the moral mission of the employer.

U Frith: I am talking about something much more concrete. Ralph Adolphs has done this. He showed people a set of 48 photographs of totally unknown faces, and they could sort them into trustworthy and non-trustworthy categories. Yet there was no objective reason for this.

Frank: Has this been shown? Is there any link between the opinion and the actual trustworthiness?

U Frith: People do tend to agree on which faces are trustworthy, but as far as I know no one has looked at the link between these opinions and actual trustworthiness. I am just saying that we are prepared to make a quick judgement, without objective evidence, on some weak signals of black and white photographs of just a face, and we agree on who is who.

Frank: I would be delighted to see whether there is any validity to the predictions.

Van Lange: Mike Kuhlmanat the University of Delaware has done some studies. There is no validity but there is some consensus. When they rate pictures, people largely agree on who is prosocial, individualist or competitive, but if you relate these judgments to the actual orientations of the people on the pictures, then you see no correlation. In other words, people agree, but they don't do better than chance in their predictions.

Gergely: I have a question about pain in rats for James Blair. Earlier you made the important point that emotions are primarily communicative. Pain is a very interesting case. The major function of pain is to avoid the source of the pain, and it may have a communicative component in so far as it is a distress call in an attachment context that helps one do that. Would you think of pain as a communicative emotion?

Blair: I don't know when rats are doing their pain sounds naturally. When Sheila King was doing her work on post-traumatic stress disorder (PTSD), she was inducing the pain in animal, but it could be that rats only express this noise when they are being eaten by something, and it is a warning to others in the group. It could have a communicatory function, but it would be surprising if it was a weird automatic noise given that all the other noises do serve some sort of purpose to provide information to close group members.

Gergely: As humans we do express vocal pain expressions, but in general we don't express emotions very much when we are alone.

Blair: I don't think anyone has shown the degree to which the pain response is modulated by the degree to which there is a person in the room. People do show emotional expressions even when they are alone, but they show them much more when they are with someone else.

Singer: Monkeys don't display a facial expression of pain.

Silk: The question of the expression of pain is enormously interesting. You have to think about what is being communicated. If expressing pain is a signal of being disabled in some way, this is very costly to display. If life is competitive and you display weakness, this is not necessarily a good thing. This needs an explanation. Primates can have hideous injuries, such as compound fracture of the femur, but although this slows them down a bit, they show very little affect of pain. When kids get injured they whimper and cry and mother picks them up. Not many other animals seem to notice, and older animals seem very stoic.

Blair: Is there a pain expressive response in chimpanzees at all? Given that these noises do tend to be communications, it is strange that they are there.

Brosnan: If it is only elicited in extreme situations it may not be meant to be a signal, but can be taken as a signal by other individuals. Just because it is a vocalization this doesn't mean it has an intended function.

Blair: I didn't imply intention, just a transmission of information.

Call: When they get hurt they will make a short scream.

Blair: Perhaps it is a warning that there is a threat stimulus in the environment.

Silk: When monkeys are threatened they often scream. This seems to be an elicitation of support.

Gergely: What about internal pain? There is no point in warning the others about a stomach ache.

Blair: I think it is just acute pain that causes these vocalizations. That's certainly the case with rats.

Brosnan: It is very difficult to determine when chimpanzees are sick or in pain. They don't act sick the way humans do and usually we cannot tell until they are quite ill.

C Frith: The fact that these might be signals puts a new light on empathy. When we show empathy it suggests that we are signalling that we are jolly nice people.

Blair: We trust people who are more expressive. They are saying that their systems are intact for being a nice human.

Blakemore: With regard to judging trustworthiness, I remember one study showing that faces of people who cooperate more in cooperative games are more memorable (Yamagishi et al 2003).

Real people played prisoner's dilemma games, and all the faces of everyone in the game were shown to a new set of subjects a year later who had no knowledge of these people. These naïve subjects did a facial memory test on these faces. Those that were more memorable were the faces of those who cooperated more. The bizarre conclusion is that people who cooperate have more memorable faces.

Singer: I have seen the paper and the effect was tiny.

Blair: That's a result that needs to be replicated.

Blakemore: You are more likely to read an email from someone with the same first name as you. Spammers have picked up on this.

Silk: It would be incredibly useful to be able to identify cooperators. In general, the problem in evolutionary theories about this is that it isn't stable because it isn't unfakeable.

Brosnan: Or that you can't fake it without a huge cost.

Silk: Yes, it has to be costly or else everyone will have that 'C' on their forehead.

Frank: I have a question for James Blair on sociopaths. There is the impression in the popular literature that they are very convincing and effective confidence tricksters who win people's trust. This seems a challenge for this account. If you could appear trustworthy and not be so, this would be the highest pay-off combination of all.

Blair: Superficial charm is one of the distinguishing features. They can be pretty effective for short periods. Having said that, there are many people who are quite easy to con. Regards the group thing, the emotion deficit does not correlate with social class, only antisocial behaviour. They do con, but it is more that healthy individuals don't like conning people in this way, such as taking an old granny's money to do roofing work and then not doing the work. It's just a bit nasty.

Frank: Would people like us be able to identify a sociopath after some interaction?

Blair: I never could.

C Frith: Let me try to say what I think I've learned from this meeting. It is clear that there is an intuitive or automatic response to other people which gives rise to emotional contagion, which may or may not be the same as empathy. This may also relate to our intuitive idea of what is fair and what is unfair. People seem to have a clear idea of this. On the other hand, people can't justify why they think things are fair or unfair. Philosophers have spent hundreds of years trying to develop schemes for classifying as things fair or unfair, but have failed. There is an interesting dichotomy here. Evolution has solved the problem, but we haven't yet. All these ideas about communication are interesting. On the one hand you automatically respond to things by changing your facial expression or behaviour, but this rapidly becomes a signal of something to other people. When it does, you can start to use it intentionally.

Sigman: There are some issues we don't all agree on. One of these is the place of affect in empathy. Is it an epiphenomenon, or a necessary part of empathy? Another issue is the direction of effects. Does it come from something implicit in the person or the other way? Is it the characteristics of the person that makes them empathic or does empathy feed back? It is interesting to see this spelled out in the economic models. What I study, I look at. Someone pretends they hurt themselves, for example, and I video the response of the autistic child. We try to code for it. Many of the children I work with have limited verbal capacity, so I have to guess from behaviour what is going on with them. The economic models are interesting, but they don't seem like what people would really do, rather more what they think about what they do.

Montague: What is the language that tells us what people would really do? What is wrong with the economic lexicon?

Sigman: I have problems with the assumption of rationality that often comes from the economic lexicon. It seems to have affected the economists themselves.

Montague: There's now a whole domain of behavioural economics that is a retreat from the rational agent model and experimental testing of it. Perhaps the economic lexicon is a bit cold. Is everything humans do in the cooperative domain living on top of some economic calculus? The one we currently have may not be close to the final form, but if we discovered that description, where would we be in all that? Is this your complaint?

Sigman: Some of it. Cold and warm are exactly the characterizations that I would use.

Montague: Suppose we discover this quantitative framework in which feeling and empathy are represented by complex equations. The fact we can do this is separate from whether or not we care about it. We can still care about having empathy and at the same time know that it is a calculus designed by a process we have no part in. Do you think that by understanding how we experience ice cream or the empathy of others, somehow its meaning will change irrevocably?

Sigman: This sort of description would be interesting, but it still might not be so compelling for me. Perhaps the most severe problem I deal with is when, for example, a mother pretends she has hurt herself and the child shows no reaction at all. Here is this whole group of people who are cut off, and you know them in 12 seconds in the elevator. They are so off, you don't even have to code their behaviour. It is such a huge difference. It would be interesting to know where this came from. I would like to be able to understand what has gone wrong.

Montague: Perhaps by disconnecting empathy from our description of it we can clear our heads a bit and see it from another point of view. It is a mechanism that was built over a long time and is very cold. It gives individuals the capacity to feel pain but it doesn't 'care'. Until we have good quantitative descriptions we are left almost completely dependent on the experts. It is hard for me to say anything sensible about autism because I don't work with it and don't have all these intuitive structures in my head like the experts. If it could be operationalized a bit then the problem could be parsed out. This is why I favour operationalization and I don't think we'd lose empathy just because we can describe it in an equation.

Sigman: It's not so much the description but the operationalization that sometimes seems to me to be far removed from what goes on.

Blair: I thought that your concern wasn't so much operationalizing the phenomenon versus not—if we could get to it we'd all use a mathematical formula. Your real concern seemed to be that some of the economic models appear to be incomplete. They look cold because they are not pulling in affect. Or they are just wrong. I don't think any of us would not want the maths if it was available to be had.

Montague: There's a fear here. If we explain everything all the way up, to why you love your children and why you like chocolate ice cream, then what is left? It removes humanity a bit. I can still care about it, though, whether or not I can write an equation about it.

Sigman: It isn't that. If we could explain everything this might give us ways to intervene.

Montague: Where do you think the economic descriptions are lacking?

Sigman: When the autistic kids are successful in social situations, it is because they worked it out cognitively, and they look like they are solving maths problems. These aren't things that most people do cognitively.

Singer: I think this debate is based on a slight misunderstanding. It seems that cognition is associated with being based on rationality and equation, whereas affective processing is emotional and is not relying on any kind of equations. Taking a computational perspective of the brain means that every process taking place in the brain is based on some sorts of computations, whether these processes are emotional or cognitive in nature.

C Frith: This is really what the meeting is about: we are trying to put the affect and the economic models together. Have we succeeded?

Silk: No, because we have attended to the problem of what it is for. Until there is more meeting of the minds about what it is for, it is going to be hard to build a good model.

Brosnan: I don't think we are going to get what it is for until we have a more operationalized definition of the characteristics we are looking for. Part of what it is for is evolutionary trajectory, and it is difficult to apply to other species in particular without this definition.

Blair: It feels as if it is massively dissociable. There are multiple systems. An argument based around a single 'for'-ness would be an unwise course of action. We'd need to do this for each system.

Warneken: It has been proposed here that economics and research focusing on affective components should be brought together, but another door that has been opened in our discussions is that of bringing together the behavioural aspects and the motivational ones. Perhaps it is not sufficient to go one *or* the other way.

Reference

Yamagishi T, Tanida S, Mashima R, Shimoma E, Kanazawa S 2003 You can judge a book by its cover: Evidence that cheaters may look different from cooperators. Evol Human Behav 24:290–301

Contributor index

Subject index